One Cause,
Many Ailments

One Cause, Many Ailments

The Leaky Gut Syndrome
What It Is and How It May Be Affecting Your Health

by
Award-winning Author
Dr. John O.A. Pagano
Chiropractic Physician

Foreword by
Harry K. Panjwani, M.D., Ph.D.

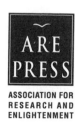

ARE PRESS

ASSOCIATION FOR
RESEARCH AND
ENLIGHTENMENT

A.R.E. Press • Virginia Beach • Virginia

DISCLAIMER

Pagano, John O.A.
    One cause—many ailments : the leaky gut syndrome : what it is and how it may be affecting your health / by Dr. John O.A. Pagano ; foreword by Harry K. Panjwani.
        p.   cm.
    Includes bibliographical references
    ISBN 978-0-87604-573-2 (trade pbk.)
    1. Intestines—Diseases—Alternative treatment. 2. Intestines—Permeability—Popular works. 3. Cayce, Edgar, 1877–1945. I. Title.
    RC806.P34 2008
    616.3′4—dc22

                                                    2008009026

A.R.E. Press
215 67th Street
Virginia Beach, VA 23451–2061

Edgar Cayce Readings © 1971, 1993–2007
by the Edgar Cayce Foundation.
All rights reserved.

Cover design by Richard Boyle

To
The memory of
Edgar Cayce

And to
Marjorie May

"Disease has changed little—
their names,
their classifications,
much!"

Edgar Cayce Reading 2002-1

CONTENTS

Foreword

Modern medicine has made major strides especially since World War II. Innovative surgical procedures using space-age technology, timely treatment of injury, burns, and accidents have reduced infections, saved lives, and hastened recovery times. Yet we have a tendency to assume that new treatments replace old treatments completely. Not so! Penicillin and aspirin will always be excellent and inexpensive drugs. For my personal oral and dental hygiene I use products made from the Neem tree of India, the use of which goes back 5000 years. In the same vein, the Yew tree, found in the northwest United States, is the source of a drug used for treatment of cancer of the ovary.

In our highly organized society, a doctor, lawyer, pilot, engineer, accountant, has to be licensed by the state for protection of citizens. With stringent protocols, continued education and on-going scrutiny by professional societies and licensing boards, a professional person has to explain and document the validity of his procedures. We have medical doctors, osteopaths, naturopaths, chiropractors, podiatrists, dieticians, nutritionists, psychologists, acupuncturists, etc., each claiming his unique skills and importance to health care.

History is replete with snake oil practitioners, and many modern day imposters often go undetected. Nevertheless, there have always been persons with God-given special unexplained gifts who heal or reduce suffering in ways which the laws of physics cannot explain. Such a person was Edgar Cayce (1877–1945).

Cayce diagnosed and gave healing suggestions to thousands of patients with varied disorders while in an altered state of consciousness, keeping meticulous records, and often offering unusual treatments. At the end of his 45 years of providing such information, his accuracy has been determined to be 93%. Yet, he was not a physician or health-care provider.

Dr. John Pagano has previously written books on psoriasis and diet based on the study of Edgar Cayce. His newest addition deals with Leaky Gut Syndrome, known professionally as *Intestinal Permeability*. Leaky Gut Syndrome does not appear as such in standard medical reference books such as the Merck Manual and/or the Physician's Desk Reference. Due to lack of clarity and interest, this problem has been overlooked by orthodox medicine.

The unusual but proven gift of Edgar Cayce combined with the lifelong commitment and dedication of Dr. Pagano to interpret his works have prompted the publication of this book. I am sure there will be skeptics. However, the reader should approach this information, which is well researched and clearly written, with an open mind and determine its suitability on an individual basis.

Some disorders, not unlike consumer products which are well-promoted and marketed, need a sponsor. Ambiguous medical problems need education, research, proper diagnosis, appropriate treatment and an open mind towards new approaches. Major supporters of medical research are pharmaceutical companies, who, understandably, would not be interested. Diseases common amongst the poor and illiterate minorities are also thus overlooked. Universities seek out research projects where there is ample funding and public demand or the involvement of high profile celebrities.

Orphan diseases need recognition, and sometimes people outside mainstream medicine have a lot to offer. Such a person is Dr. Pagano!

Harry K. Panjwani, M.D., Ph.D.
December 2007

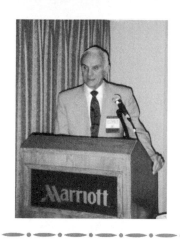

Preface

What is it that arthritis, chronic fatigue, migraine headaches, celiac disease, psoriasis, diabetes, lupus, as well as many other diseases, have in common? At first glance they appear to be totally unrelated, yet, in the light of present day knowledge, they may very well be linked by a common denominator, hidden from view, but nevertheless held suspect as an underlying factor in many of mankind's physical and even mental ailments.

I refer to a condition that probably existed since the dawn of history but was unrecognized until now: *Intestinal Permeability* or the *Leaky Gut Syndrome (LGS)*. The name is a perfect description of what can and does happen within our intestinal tract that manifests itself in a number of ailments that mankind is heir to. That's the bad news. The good news is that these seemingly insurmountable problems can be helped, alleviated, and in many cases healed. Once the underlying cause of a problem is recognized, one can proceed to correct the situation in an intelligent, reasonable manner rather than in a haphazard "hit or miss" way. It puts a handle on things. You know what you are doing, and more important, you know why you are doing it.

The purpose of this volume is to shed more light on the subject based on experience rather than on theory or speculation. Evidence of the efficacy of this approach will be included in this work. A picture is still worth a thousand words, so I make use of illustrations and before-and-after photos to substantiate my claims. Having authored two books on the subject and having lectured on five continents about psoriasis and eczema using the concept of the "leaky gut" as the basis of my approach, I felt honored and deeply moved when Charles Thomas Cayce, President of the A.R.E., Virginia Beach, Virginia, called in March of 2006 and asked that I write a book on this subject since so many letters and reports came in over the years proving how effective and satisfying this approach has been to the many sufferers of these two diseases.

Without question I look upon the Leaky Gut Syndrome as the underlying culprit behind many of the diseases known to man. These illnesses will remain his legacy until the basic causes are recognized, addressed, and removed. Fortunately there are answers and remedies for such a condition that may astonish you. It is my purpose to reveal those answers as I have experienced and witnessed them, and prove to those who have eyes to see and ears to hear, that Intestinal Permeability, or a Leaky Gut, is something to be taken seriously and not brushed aside as an interesting but unimportant theory–and that therapy of certain diseases will not necessarily begin on the end organ affected, but on the *origin* of the problem, namely, in many cases, the Leaky Gut.

Dr. John O.A. Pagano
Englewood Cliffs, N.J.
October 2007

PART I
The Leaky Gut Syndrome (LGS)
Intestinal Permeability

1

——•——•——•——•——•——•——

The Anatomy of the Disease

What is meant by a "leaky gut" anyway? We've heard of a broken leg, a bleeding ulcer, a ruptured appendix, a torn ligament—but a leaky gut? Who ever heard of it? If it has been known in the field of gastroenterology I'd say it is one of their best kept secrets. It is anything but a household word, yet, as this elusive disease (or condition) has slowly come into focus as a possible cause of many other conditions, new light has been shed on health problems that heretofore were considered "unknown" or "incurable" when it came to origins.

Upon hearing the term for the first time, many of us may have visions of blood, lymph, body fluids, etc. seeping through the stomach wall and flooding the entire abdominal cavity. Such is not the case. Clearly, it is the exact opposite. The "leak" we speak of goes *from* the abdominal cavity *into* the blood, not from the blood into the abdominal cavity. The reason for this will become clear to you as we proceed.

I suppose it is only natural when you have a persistent headache, you hold your head with the idea that the problem starts in your head. In some cases, that is, of course, true, but more often than not the culprit lies elsewhere. I can't count the number of times in my practice

1

when a chronic, persistent headache has finally been relieved by a simple home enema, the patient having suffered from a fecal impaction in the colon. In other cases, a long-standing problem with headache dissipated with a change in diet! The patient was allergic to certain foods that he didn't realize until he avoided them.

In another dramatic case, excruciating pain persisted down a patient's left arm that seemed to originate from the left side of his cervical spine (neck). He could not sleep or function because of the great discomfort he was experiencing. All my testing indicated that he had a condition known as brachial neuritis originating in the 5th, 6th and 7th cervical vertebrae. I used every means at my disposal—electrotherapy, ultrasound, adjustments—but nothing seemed to work. I was at my wits end when the patient went to see his dentist for a problem he was having with a tooth.

This proved to be a godsend, for the dentist discovered an abscessed molar of long standing on the left side of his jaw. The dentist extracted the infected tooth, and my patient reported that the stench of infection was so pungent that the doctor and his assistant had to leave the room and open windows to air out the office. The area of the extraction was then cleaned and disinfected. Relief of my patient's arm pain was immediate! No more neck pain, no more arm pain, only blessed relief— "God blessed relief"—is how my patient expressed it.

Of course, there is a scientific explanation of why such results were obtained, but the fact is that the patient didn't care, the doctor didn't care—the job was done and nothing else mattered.

The list could go on and on, but the essence of what I am saying is that the origin of many diseases may not be so obvious at first glance— that is why I look upon the leaky gut as an elusive disease. You can't see it; it is hidden from view, pain may or may not be present, and unless special tests such as gastroscope testing, or even biopsy of the gut wall is medically performed, it may remain unrecognized and continue to evade the diagnostician.

The Leaky Gut Syndrome Defined

"The official definition of the Leaky Gut is an increase in permeability

of the intestinal mucosa to luminal macromolecules, antigens and toxins associated with inflammatory degenerative and/or atrophic mucosal damage." (AIA Newsletter, 1997)

In 1995 Dr. Zoltan Rona, M.D., M.Sc, of Toronto, Canada, author of
several health books, wrote a short, concise discourse on the leaky gut
that I found to be right to the point in describing this medical phenomenon. I take this quotation from my book *Healing Psoriasis: The Natural
Alternative*:

> The Leaky Gut Syndrome is the name given to a very common
> health disorder in which the basic organic defect [lesion] is an
> *intestinal lining* which is more permeable [porous] than nor-
> mal. The abnormally large spaces present between the cells
> of the gut wall allow the entry of toxic material into the blood-
> stream that would, in healthier circumstances, be repelled and
> eliminated. The gut becomes leaky in the sense that bacteria,
> fungi, parasites and their toxins, undigested protein, fat and
> waste normally not absorbed into the bloodstream in the
> healthy state, pass through a damaged, hyperpermeable, po-
> rous, or leaky gut.

I found it fascinating to read a similar description of the mechanism
involved by Edgar Cayce, in his discourses made in 1944, about a woman
suffering from psoriasis, in reading 3373–1:

> There are disturbing conditions which prevent the better
> physical functioning in this body. These have to do primarily
> with an *intestinal disorder* and the lack of proper coordination
> in the eliminating systems. There are those conditions, then,
> in the duodenum and through the jejunum where there are
> the effects as if there were tiny thinned walls, as if the walls of
> the duodenum had been smoothed—rather than the folds
> that should exist with the gastric flow which should come
> through these areas at periods of digestion. The results are a
> disturbance in the blood supply and an irritation in the super-
> ficial circulation, so that those areas in the epidermis show
> eliminations that should be carried through [the] alimentary
> canal, for these are being eliminated through [the] perspira-
> tory system.

When one dissects the wording of reading 3373-1 it is obvious that Cayce was describing what is now known as the leaky gut. Although not identified as such at the time of the reading, it most certainly bears all the earmarks of this now recognized disease entity. How he was able to do that is the reason the ever popular television program *Unsolved Mysteries* as well as the History Channel saw fit to bring it to the screen and feature Cayce's story around the world. Nevertheless, the foremost question is: Was it true or was it false? And if it is true, how was Edgar Cayce able to tap into this knowledge and bring it into the world? Or could it be that there are, in fact, mysteries in this world that we earthlings are unaware of? (But that would be the subject of another book!)

In *The Maker's Diet*, author Jordan Rubin quotes the following statement made by Dr. H.H. Boeker in 1928: "It is now universally conceded that autointoxication is the underlying cause of an exceptionally large group of symptom complexes. Recent research seems to support these earlier conclusions about intestinal toxemia. Yet, many modern medical practitioners and researchers still dismiss intestinal toxemia as a concept that is 'old and outdated'." (Rubin, 2004–05, p. 57)

Rubin continues the Dr. Boeker statement " . . . 90 percent of diseases are caused or complicated by toxins created in the intestinal tract by unhealthy foods that are not properly eliminated. Autointoxication occurs when, due to poor elimination, certain toxins escape from the bowel into the blood stream and poison the body, causing a silent form of self-poisoning." (Rubin, 2004–05, p. 58)

Could there be a more perfect description of the leaky gut syndrome than that? As early as 1928 (perhaps earlier) such a disease entity has been recognized by renowned physicians, such as Dr. Boeker, but largely ignored by the "scientific" community.

Be that as it may. I had reason to prove it with my first psoriasis patient, Mr. William Culmone, in 1975 when he came into my office with a low back problem (permission to use his full name has been granted). When he disrobed for me to examine his spine it startled me to see that he had another problem as well—psoriasis! Psoriasis is but one of the many diseases which is suspected to originate from a leaky gut.

Since I was already into the study of psoriasis, not only from a medical perspective, but from the discourses of Edgar Cayce himself, it occurred to me to ask Mr. Culmone if he would be interested in experimenting with me after clearing up his back problem. His answer was "Why not? I tried everything else for fifteen years!"

Once the low back cleared up, we began our "research." Since all the measures called for in the Cayce discourses on psoriasis fell within the scope of my chiropractic practice, I felt justified in giving it a try, especially since the patient was fully cooperative. Following the basic concept of the leaky gut as the culprit in such cases we proceeded to follow the suggestions that might possibly bring about a healing of this dermatological enigma.

It wasn't long before Mr. Culmone showed signs of improvement. In fact, within seven days the heavy, thick lesions on his back and thighs were reduced by at least fifty percent! Within the following three months, all lesions disappeared. He remained free of all signs of psoriasis for the rest of his life.

It became very clear from the outset of the regimen *that diet played the key role.* Why? Because of the beneficial effect a change of diet had on the irritated walls of his small intestine. To a large degree he avoided fats (especially from red meat), inflammatory foods such as the Nightshades, too many sweets, and fried foods, among others. As stated earlier, the results were startling. He was my first case in which I approached the problem using the theory of a compromised intestinal lining. The success achieved set me on a course of therapy, at least in psoriasis and eczema, for over forty years, and continues to this day.

All other measures, i.e., oils, herb teas, spinal adjustments, steam baths, etc., played an important but relatively secondary role. Often when I lecture, I tell my audience that "I have never helped, alleviated, or improved one case of psoriasis on a patient who did not follow the diet." Yet, there are hundreds, if not thousands, of people who achieved what may be called "miraculous" results by doing it on their own simply by following the suggestions in my books *Healing Psoriasis: The Natural Alternative* and *Dr. John's Healing Psoriasis Cookbook . . . Plus!* Impartial evidence of this can be found by logging on to Amazon.com, typing in "healing psoriasis," and reading over fifty book reviews by people who did it on their own; people I have never seen!

Further evidence of cases of psoriasis and eczema will be presented as we proceed. The point to grasp here is that if such a protocol can work on cases of psoriasis, a condition that has plagued mankind since the dawn of history and is still considered medically incurable, what can it do for other conditions that are equally devastating to suffering humanity? I submit that taking a hard look at such a possibility is indeed justified!

If, for example, as medical literature suggests, multiple sclerosis (MS) may possibly be linked to a leaky gut, then why not consider muscular dystrophy (MD) or amyotrophic lateral sclerosis (ALS) in the same vein? Other degenerative diseases such as the devastating scleroderma may or may not have a similar origin, but is it so unreasonable to at least consider the possibility? Such a condition has already been treated successfully and documented and is available in the Cayce archives. *Here, in my humble opinion, is where extensive scientific research should be concentrated, on the degenerative diseases and their relation to intestinal permeability—or the leaky gut.* Perhaps that is what Cayce meant in his discourse 2002-1 when he said disease has changed little, but classifications, much.

2

————•————•————•————•————•————

The Anatomy Involved

Most everyone with a reasonable amount of education knows we have a mouth that leads into the esophagus, which in turn leads into the stomach, and from the stomach, the intestinal tract, and finally the large intestine, or colon. That's about it. And in most cases, that's all that's necessary to get on in this world as far as digestion is concerned. With a little bit of luck, this sequence of anatomical structures, which constitutes the alimentary canal, will serve us faithfully, if not abused over a long period of time.

But when something goes awry in any of these sections, repair begins at once and can range from natural healing to open surgery, depending on the nature of the problem. This is nothing new. But what may be considered new to most people is how these organs are put together. The cellular structure that makes up the body is mind–boggling. Since we are concerned primarily with the small intestine, let's focus on this tube that stretches from the lower end of the stomach to the ileocecal valve that leads into the five–foot–long *large intestine* (the colon) and through the sigmoid colon and rectum, where the residue of digestion exits the body.

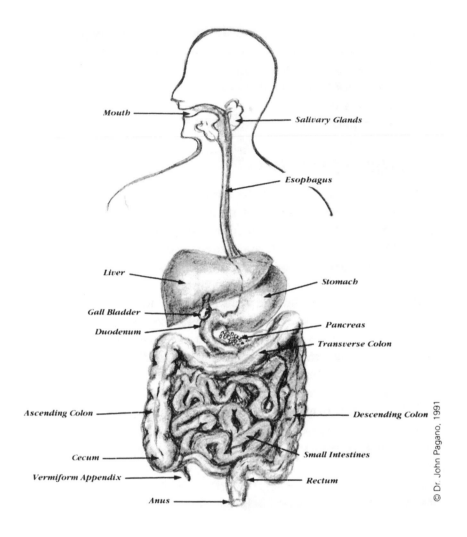

Fig. P2 — The Normal Digestive Tract

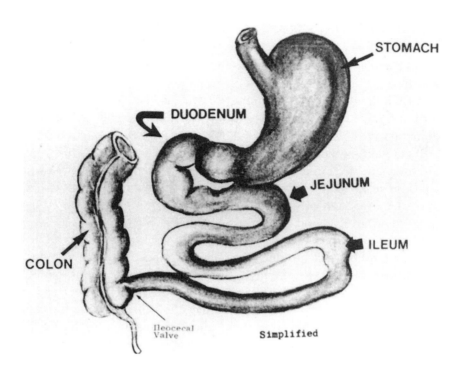

Fig. P3 — Where the Leaky Gut Begins

The Digestive Process

Food, partially digested, moves out of the stomach after it has been processed to a certain degree by enzymes and acids, and enters the first section of the small intestine known as the *duodenum*. Here it is further acted upon by body chemicals and passes on as *chyme* into the next section of the small intestine, known as the *jejunum*, where most of the transfer of nutrients takes place. The chyme then moves on into the *ileum*, the longest section of the small intestine, where more transfer of nutrients takes place and residue that is not absorbable mixes with water and waste products of digestion and moves into the *large intestine* (the colon) for evacuation from the body.

The entire length of the small intestine is approximately twenty-two to twenty-eight feet. Add to that the length of the colon, five feet, and you have an intestinal tract that is over four times the height of the average individual. If the small intestine were not designed to twist and turn and have numerous convolutions, it could never fit into the abdominal cavity.

If you take a small piece of the jejunum, the second part of the small intestine, and section a piece of it and put it under a microscope you will find innumerable structures known as *intestinal villi* that sway to and fro, like a sea of grass or an ocean wave. Their purpose is to receive nutrients from the food and drink you ingest, but they also act as a barrier for unwanted materials. Nutrients are very small (*micromolecules*) compared to the waste products (*macromolecules*) such as fat, yeast, undigested protein (peptides), germs, bacteria, etc., which are considerably larger. So the intestinal villi have a two-fold function: as a "guardian at the gate" preventing the large macromolecules from breaking through the barrier, and, at the same time, allowing the helpful nutrients, micromolecules, to pass on through to be absorbed by the lymphatic system and transferred into the bloodstream. The nutrients are then carried by way of the blood circulatory system to every cell of the body for nourishment, growth, and repair. Thus the cycle of life continually takes place.

Now that's the best case scenario. What I did not mention was that a lot can happen to that twenty-two to twenty-eight feet of intestine that is most undesirable to the living organism known as homo sapiens. It is my purpose to bring to your attention just one of those conditions affecting mankind, the knowledge of which could save him/her from ailments whose origins, heretofore, have been categorized as "unknown."

In spite of the magnificence of the structure and function of our intestinal tract, it is not immune to certain conditions that render it compromised or simply damaged. I refer to a condition known in medical circles for many years; but it is rarely given credence and is therefore often overlooked. That condition, to which any one of us is subject, is known as Intestinal Permeability, or the Leaky Gut Syndrome (LGS).

We stated earlier that the jejunum is the primary section of the small intestine where most of the nutrients pass through the walls of the intestine and enter the bloodstream, which in turn nourishes every cell (sixty trillion!) of the body. Damage to this section of the small intestine, however, will allow the larger molecules of toxins and irritants of one kind or another to pass through as well. These destructive elements pollute the bloodstream and are carried to the myriad of cells to every organ of the body where the blood goes. In other words, where the blood goes, so go the pollutants. In some cases, permeability of the large (toxic) molecules takes place while permeability of the small (nutrient) molecules is prevented, causing malabsorption and malnutrition.

So, a person may develop diabetes, for instance, because the cells of the pancreas (Islets of Langerhans) become affected by the poisoned blood. This can apply to any organ of the body, as well as the joints (arthritis), the brain (schizophrenia, mental depression), and the skin (psoriasis, eczema), among others. Admittedly this is theory—but is it really so farfetched? I think not.

If it is true that a leaky gut is the basic cause of many diseases, especially those that are degenerative, it seems to me that healing the walls of the intestines is the most logical step to follow. Can this be done? I state without reservation that it can be and has been done!

Remember that the macrovilli and microvilli of the inner wall (lumen) of the intestines number into the millions and billions, respectively. It is estimated that there are twenty thousand villi and ten billion microvilli in *one square inch* of intestinal lining! The attack (for lack of a better word) comes from the inside—or the inner wall of the intestinal tube. The way to approach a possible remedy is, consequently, from the inside. Admittedly this is not an earth–shattering concept. It's just plain common sense. The next question is: How does one do that?

The answer is twofold. First, we can put a halt to the irritants causing the problem, i.e., yeast, viruses, bacterial overload, etc., by destroying or removing them. Second, we can provide soothing, ingested remedies whose function it is to heal the inner walls of the intestines. This is the key to the healing of the disease, which is covered in Part II of this book.

The Gastro-Intestinal (GI) Tract

Without a healthy GI tract, you are always sick in one way or another—or you die! Your death may be the result of a slow, insidious process, but you will be just as dead as you would be from a speeding bullet! Therefore, it is helpful to know a little about the GI tract and how it functions. The following are the primary functions of our GI tract:

1. It digests food.
2. It absorbs small food molecules which supply the fuel and energy of the body.
3. It carries nutrients, like vitamins and minerals, which are attached to what are called *carrier proteins* across the gut wall into the bloodstream.
4. It plays a major role in detoxification of harmful chemicals in the body.
5. It fights infection through immunoglobulins (antibodies) which act as the first line of defense against infection.

No minor task you might say. Yet, in the healthy state it carries out those functions as easily as a normal person walks across the street. But, when damage exists within the GI tract, its function is impaired, not unlike that person trying to walk across the street with two sprained ankles.

That's when inflammation of the intestinal tract can cause all kinds of havoc—*anywhere* in the body! In the light of this knowledge, therefore, it seems a mistake to treat areas (or organs) of the body without giving the slightest consideration to the possibility of the GI tract being even remotely involved.

Signs of the Disease—
What Happens When the Gut Is Inflamed?

Objective Signs

When changes in the lining of the intestinal tract take place, there are certain telltale signs that offer a clue that the patient may be suffering from a leaky gut, causing toxic elements to invade the blood stream.

Objective signs (observed by someone other than the patient) include everything from skin rash of one kind or another, bloating of the stomach, and impaired growth (as in the case of celiac disease) to malaise, malnutrition, nasal coryza (as in the case of allergic sensitivity), mucous stools (as in the case of irritable bowel syndrome, IBS), as well as blood in the stools (as in the case of parasite infection).

Subjective Signs

Subjective signs (experienced by the patient) carry a wide variety of symptoms, such as: pain in the stomach and intestinal area (especially upon palpation of these areas), pain in the joints and spine, chronic constipation and/or diarrhea, headache, attention deficit, skin disease, hyperactive or under-active behavior, fever, altered blood sugar levels contributing to diabetes, toxic liver symptoms, allergies, asthma, and a myriad of other symptoms.

Dr. Leo Galland, M.D., gastroenterologist, director of the Foundation for Integrated Medicine, and author of *Power Healing*, is one of the foremost authorities on the leaky gut. The following list of symptoms associated with increased intestinal permeability is taken directly from his informative online article "Leaky Gut Syndromes: Breaking the Vicious Cycle" (www.mdheal.org/leakygut.htm).

Symptoms Associated with Increased Intestinal Permeability:

Fatigue and malaise	Diarrhea
Arthralgias	Skin rashes
Myalgias	Toxic feelings
Fevers of unknown origin	Cognitive and memory deficits
Food intolerances	Shortness of breath
Abdominal pain	Poor exercise tolerance
Abdominal distension	

Dr. Galland goes on to say in the same article "Unless specifically investigated, the role of altered intestinal permeability in patients with Leaky Gut Syndrome often goes unrecognized."

The Seven Stages of the Inflamed Gut

The seven stages of the 'inflamed' gut, according to the AIA Newsletter (1997), are as follows:

1. When the gut is inflamed, it does not absorb nutrients and foods properly and so fatigue and bloating can occur.

2. As mentioned previously, when large food particles are absorbed there is the creation of food allergies and new symptoms with target organs, such as, arthritis or fibromyalgia.

3. When the gut is inflamed the carrier proteins are damaged so nutrient deficiencies occur which can also cause any symptom, like magnesium deficiency induced muscle spasm or copper deficiency induced high cholesterol. [Author's note: or gold–deficiency–induced multiple sclerosis, covered later in this book.]

4. Likewise, when the detox pathways that line the gut are compromised, chemical sensitivity can arise. Furthermore, the leakage of toxins overburdens the liver so that the body is less able to handle everyday chemicals.

5. When the gut lining is inflamed the protective coating of IgA (immunoglobulin A) is adversely affected and the body is not able to ward off protozoa, bacteria, viruses and yeasts like candida.

6. When the intestinal lining is inflamed, bacteria and yeasts are able to translocate. This means they are able to pass from the gut lumen or cavity, into the bloodstream and set up infection anywhere else in the body.

7. The worst symptom is the formation of antibodies. Sometimes these leak across and look similar to antigens on our own tissues. Consequently, when an antibody is made to attack it, it also attacks our tissue. This is probably how autoimmune diseases start. Rheumatoid arthritis, lupus, multiple sclerosis, thyroiditis and many others are members of this ever–growing category of "incurable" diseases." (AIA Newsletter, 1997)

3

———•———•———•———•———

Causes of LGS

What Causes the Breakdown of the Intestinal Walls?

We know now that the inner walls (lumen) of the intestinal tract can break down to such an extent that macro (large) molecules of one type or another pass through this natural barrier and travel, along with the smaller molecular nutrients, and deposit in the blood stream via the lymphatic channels located in the walls of the microvilli of the villi.

But, what is it that destroys these walls? Get the answer to that and you have half the solution on correcting the problem, if possible. That it *is* possible is not so remote. The inner lumen has remarkable regenerative powers. It is the most recuperative of any organ in the body by virtue of the fact that it has a very rich blood supply that allows it to renew itself every three to six days. This is a physiological fact. The question then is why doesn't it repair itself routinely in cases of leaky gut? As long as the irritant(s) continue to be present, it cannot repair itself. The first counterattack to the problem, therefore, is to identify the culprit(s). Once it is determined, remove it or stop it in its tracks. *Just that*

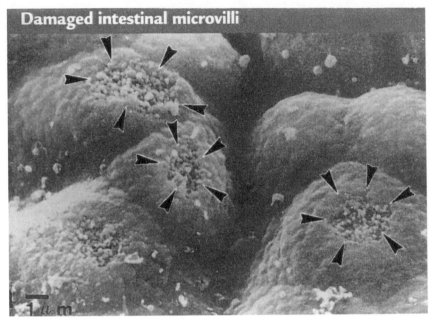

Fig. P4 — Damaged Intestinal Microvilli
[Reproduced through the courtesy of the Genova Diagnostic Lab]

action alone may solve a major part of the healing process. Whether the break-down is due to destructive organisms (like yeasts), too many antibiotics, a poor diet (you may be eating *good* food—but for you it may be the *wrong* food!) will determine the course of action to take in resolving the problem.

It has been my experience, after being in clinical practice for nearly half a century, that in many cases, it is what the patient *stays away from* that brings about a healing. I am convinced that this is the case when it comes to hyperpermeable intestinal damage—or the Leaky Gut.

What Causes the Gut to Leak?

We have listed many aspects of LGS, from what happens when the gut leaks, signs and symptoms, definitions, etc. That is all well and good—but one aspect of the condition remains which must be understood. What causes the pinholes to occur in the first place? The leaky gut may be the cause of the various diseases, *but what causes the leaky gut?*

There is a very helpful Web site, www.candidafree.net, maintained by Mark and Alyson Cobb. On their site, they inform us of a Dr. William Cowden, a physician who studied the underlying cause of many diseases, who determined that a major etiology of many diseases is an *overgrowth of candida albicans*, or simply *candida*.

Here's how it works. A yeast build-up forms within the folds of the small intestine. Since these are very prolific, they will continue to grow within the villi and microvilli of the intestinal walls. It is true that yeast is normally found in the intestines, but when they are allowed to grow undisturbed, the yeast begins to morph and forms a fungus deep in the folds of the intestines. They make a "home" there so to speak, and settle in. The fungus then forms roots, like a plant, called *rhizoids*. These rhizoids eventually actually penetrate the intestinal walls, and in so doing, they form the holes which characterize the leaky gut—thus the yeast/fungal overgrowth of candida. The rhizoids continue their growth through the walls of the intestine in their quest for blood and the glucose it contains, which is needed to feed the yeast. This process is not unlike the roots of a tree that grow deep in the ground, much longer and more extended than the tree itself, in search of water. The result is the Leaky Gut Syndrome. Therefore, the most effective way to control, alleviate or even cure the disease is to destroy the yeast overgrowth or flush it out of the system.

The Cause of the Perforations— The Yeast-Fungi-Mold Connection

We have learned that the fungus formed by yeast overgrowth is one of the major causes of the breakdown of the intestinal wall as mentioned earlier. *The fungus grows roots that eventually penetrate the intestinal walls, thereby forming the holes that allow the toxic elements of bacteria, viruses, undigested protein, acids, and numerous other waste products to gain passage through the natural barrier and enter the* lymphatic system.

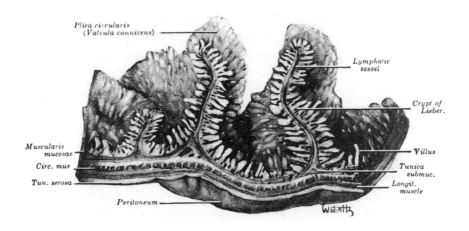

Fig. P5—Cross-section of Intestinal Villi from Gray's Anatomy
This demonstrates the many crevasses where yeast
may collect and continue to grow undisturbed.
Gray's Anatomy (26th ed. Philadelphia, Lea and Febiger, 1954.
30th Ed., Pub. 1985, Carmine D. Clemente, Ed.)

The lymphatic system dumps into the blood circulatory system primarily through the thoracic duct, the lymphatic system's main trunk
which lies along the spine, and enters a large vein on the left, close to
the heart, thus establishing the pollution of the blood stream.

We are dealing with infected or polluted blood and lymph. Blood, as
you well know, goes everywhere. In fact, if *any* organ or cell is deprived
of blood, that organ or cell malfunctions, deteriorates, and eventually
dies. By *everywhere* I mean exactly that—from the largest organ of the
body, the skin, which in the average adult measures about eighteen
square feet, to the tiniest microcells of the brain and spinal cord. Symptoms of every description can soon become apparent, thus the reason
for the many seemingly different diseases previously listed as having
an inflamed, damaged, or leaky gut as their origin.

Please understand, I am not implying that all diseases are caused by
a leaky gut. What I am saying is that it can be a major *basic underlying
cause* of many, especially the chronic degenerative diseases. Perhaps

more important is the fact that it is rarely taken into consideration by the attending physician. He/she will run every test imaginable to assess the cause of the patient's problem—from blood tests, x–rays, CT scans, MRIs, isotrophic testing, sound, and mental evaluation, etc., etc., etc. But how often does a physician order a simple, inexpensive Intestinal Permeability test (lactulose/mannitol challenge)? The answer is *hardly ever!* And if the doctor has never *heard* of the test, he cannot order it. (More on this test is featured later.)

In my opinion, any physician who orders such a test when LGS is suspected is doing his patient a great service. Even if it comes back negative, at least it will give the attending doctor an indication of what may be ruled out.

I end this section with a quote from the works of Edgar Cayce when he was asked if there was an absolute cure for psoriasis (which was due to a leaky gut). His answer was:

> Most of this is found in diet. There is a cure. It requires patience, persistence, and right thinking also.   2455-2

In my opinion, this short passage is Cayce's great gift to all psoriasis and eczema patients everywhere and may very well apply to all cases in which a leaky gut is found to be the origin. In a few words he gives the answer to its remedy "most of this is found in diet." He offers hope that "there is a cure," and then adds what it will cost: "patience, persistence" and to top it off, "right thinking."

Simple? Undoubtedly! Easy? Not necessarily! The attitude of the patient and those around him plays a significant role. It is not easy to change a lifestyle, especially as it relates to diet. Then there are others who would welcome a diet designed to rid their body of this devastating disease. It all goes back to priorities. "Do you want to get rid of the problem, or don't you?" is a question I ask of patients, new ones in particular. Their answer to that one question will determine their future.

Specific Causes

After many years of research and observation, the scientific community has come up with a number of potential irritants that may play a role in developing a damaged intestinal inner wall. The following are a few that are listed in the Functional Assessment Resource Manual of the Genova (formerly Great Smokies) Diagnostic Laboratory:

Nonsteroidal anti-inflammatory drugs (NSAID)
HIV infection
Intestinal Infection
Maldigestion / Malabsorption
Alcoholism
Aging
Deficient SLGA
Giardiasis
Ingestion of allergic foods
Ingestion of offending chemicals
Trauma and endotoxins
(Ball, Runkel and Holmes, 1999, pG–31)

Having dealt with the subject for many years, I feel compelled to add my "two cents worth" to this list of substances that cause damage to the intestinal mucosa. By practical experience I include in this list of culprits:

1. A poor diet over a long period of time: one that is high in acidic reactions, saturated fats, inflammatory foods such as the nightshades (covered later), yeast, grains and sugars

2. Stress factors

3. Spinal subluxations, especially areas of the 5th through the 9th thoracic vertebrae (See Chapter 5, The Spinal Connection.)

4. Negative emotions, harbored resentments

5. Chronic constipation

6. Too many sweets

7. Fried foods

8. Smoking

9. Alcohol

10. Transmission of toxins by the mother in the case of the newborn

Read the above lists. Does any item ring a bell in your mind? The chances are you will find one or more that stand out as something that applies to you. Take heed to it, for therein may lie your antagonist when it comes to food selection. *Remember, he is a fool who thinks the nutritional value of a food is determined by its taste!*

Nonsteroidal Anti-Inflammatory Drugs (NSAID)

Dr. Leo Galland, Dr. Zoltan Rona, Dr. Andrew Weil, and the Genova Diagnostic Laboratory Functional Assessment Resource Manual, as well as many other renowned researchers, list nonsteroidal anti-inflammatory drugs (NSAIDs) and overuse of antibiotics as a primary cause of the breakdown of the intestinal walls. These painkillers are prescribed especially in the treatment of chronic arthritic pain.

You would think that drugs are the answer when an overgrowth of pathogens, especially bacteria, viruses, and germs, are part of the problem of LGS. The fact is antibiotics kill *all* the bacteria in the intestines, not just the bad guys. There are innumerable bacteria throughout the intestinal tract—both good and bad. The trick is to be sure the good (friendly) bacteria dominate the bad ones at all times. This is called *symbiosis*. If this ratio is reversed, all sorts of havoc takes place throughout the intestinal tract. This is referred to as *dysbiosis;* they just don't balance out right.

"Balancing out right" does not mean a ratio of 50/50. Remember, the friendly bacteria must override the bad ones by a large margin, or you are in trouble. This is not unlike the "normal" ratio of acid and alkaline foods that will be discussed in Part II of this book. Normal in the acid/alkaline balance of foods does not mean 50/50 either. Rather it means 70–80 percent alkaline formers to 20–30 percent acid formers. The difference is as crucial in food selection as it is in friendly bacteria and bad bacteria in the GI tract. That ratio distinguishes an unhealthy gut from a healthy one. When the proper balance is established, everybody gets along, harmony sets in, and symbiosis is the end result.

4

—•—•—•—•—•—

What to Do About It?

re there answers to healing the leaky gut? Well, yes and no! This is
not playing with words—it is an unmitigated statement of fact.
There are answers as to how to heal the compromised gut wall. The
question is, however, *will the patient follow through?*

Remember, according to most authorities, the inner lining of the intestinal mucosa regenerates itself about once a week. Therefore, we can
assume it has remarkable healing powers, but, as mentioned previously,
unless the irritant (whatever it may be) is removed from the scene, the
cells of the villi and microvilli cannot heal. Consequently, through self-
evaluation and the help of the patient's personal physician, more often
than not, one can figure out the cause of the problem.

The first thing I question my patients about is their diet. I seek out what
their *favorite* foods are. In a majority of cases, I find that they not only
like certain foods, they *gorge* themselves on them! What they do not
know is that their favorite foods may be the foods that are tearing their guts
apart. Literally! The greatest offenders will be covered later in this book.

Another question I ask my patients is whether or not they have been
on drugs (prescription or otherwise) for any extended period of time.

Another is whether or not the patient is a smoker or drinker, or both! In other words, do they consume too many gut irritants, and if so, for how long have they been doing it?

Here is what the questions should focus on. Once discovered and addressed, there is a good chance that the healing process can start. Again, the trick is to *follow through*. Avoid items that cause the breakdown, especially free radicals, consume those that built it up, such as antioxidants, and then—*give time a chance!* Like anything else, the patient must be committed. He cannot play at it and expect results.

[Author's Note: The author recognizes the fact that the above explanation is relatively simple in its content. He also acknowledges the fact that many of his readers insist upon a more scientific, detailed explanation. For those who fall into this category, he enthusiastically refers them to the impressive work of Leo Galland, M.D., director of the Foundation of Integrative Medicine. His in-depth discourse "Leaky Gut Syndromes: Breaking the Vicious Cycle" can be downloaded from his Web site: www.mdheal.org/leakygut.htm.]

A Helpful Analogy

It may be helpful to consider the following analogy. You may compare your damaged intestinal villi to a neglected lawn. Grass cannot grow because it is being choked off by weeds, debris, stones, and all manner of things that prevent nutrition from reaching the roots of each blade of grass. Before long the grass withers, dries up, and dies.

But if the caretaker rakes the lawn, pulls the weeds, and picks up the dead leaves and debris, he will be preparing the land for the next step, re-seeding. He will then scatter the new seed and add nutrients to the soil. With regular watering, new sprouts will begin to show. Then he maintains the lawn with proper watering and regular care to keep the weeds and other destructive elements under control. All things being equal, a new lawn will beautify his property.

In essence, repairing a damaged, compromised gut wall is a similar process, only this time the blades of grass are the millions upon millions of microscopic villi that line the lumen of the intestinal tract. All in all, that twenty-two to twenty-eight feet of small intestines, if spread out, would cover the same area as a tennis court! The weeds, debris, stones, and dead leaves which cut off the normal elements (including sunlight) that provide growth, are analogous to the destructive elements that coat the deep recesses of the villi and microvilli. These deleterious elements are *yeast* and *fungi* in particular, but include bacteria, germs, viruses, fats, acids, undigested protein, and anything else the host consumes that can clog the junction of where the villi meet the intestinal wall. When this happens a slow, but steady, deterioration of the gut wall takes place.

To complete the analogy, the re-seeding of the internal lawn of the intestinal wall takes place when the probiotics (L. acidophilus and B. bifidus) are ingested and these good bacteria grow and populate the intestinal wall, overwhelming and replacing the bad bacteria and bringing about a state of symbiosis. The watering of the internal lawn occurs through the intake of large quantities of pure water that flush the toxic elements out of the system.

The problem is one doesn't really know that the pathologic process is taking place since initially there are few, if any, warning signs. It is not until the end organ, i.e., the area infected, raises its head by one symptom or another clueing you in to the fact that something is amiss. It may be an effect upon the eyes and vision, it may be irritable bowel syndrome (IBS) or Crohn's disease, an inflammation at the junction of the small intestine and the large bowel (ileocecal valve), asthma (the lungs), migraine headaches, skin diseases like psoriasis or eczema, celiac disease—first recognized in young children who do not grow and have a bulbous abdomen. (See my chapter on Celiac Disease.) Whatever it is, it may very well be due to a gut that leaks toxins into the bloodstream which in turn travels throughout the body in search of a weak spot to muscle in on and take over, so to speak.

We have just covered what causes the perforations that take place in the gut wall. Knowing that answers a great many questions. This is, of course, the most important aspect of this study, for it not only provides us with a cause of the disease, but the solution as well.

To summarize, the scientific procedure that we have described is known as the "4 Rs"—Remove—Replace—Reinoculate—Repair. Each of these will be covered in Part II of this book.

5

—•—•—•—•—•—•—•—

The Spinal Connection

Of all the references that give reasons for the breakdown of the intestinal walls, I know of only one that recognizes the role of spinal misalignments (subluxations)—the Edgar Cayce readings, specifically readings 4000–1 and 4001–1.

Here we learn for the first time that there is a spinal connection that can, and probably often does, play a part in the integrity of the intestinal walls as they relate to the leaky gut. It is a matter of basic anatomy and physiology.

Reading 4000–1 states in part:

> . . . there is somewhat of a complication of disturbances. These arise primarily from a subluxation existing in the upper dorsal areas which in the beginning or in times back slowed the circulation through the abdominal areas.
>
> Thus we have an impoverishment to the alimentary canal— a thinning of the walls. This allowed the circulation to draw, through absorption, the alimentary canal poisons which accumulate in the lymph producing great splotches—first as pimples and then red, scaly blotches that cause disfigurement

and aggravation to the body. To correct the situation, we first give the body some eight to ten spinal adjustments, especially the 5th and 6th dorsal vertebrae and also align or coordinate the lumbar and sacral area.

(Author's note: A "subluxation" is a vertebra out of its normal alignment that affects the nerve[s] emitting from between vertebrae. The above reading mentions the 5th and 6th dorsal vertebrae; however, most of the readings center on the 6th and 7th dorsal for the leaky gut. I personally adjust the 5th through 9th dorsal region and balance it out.)

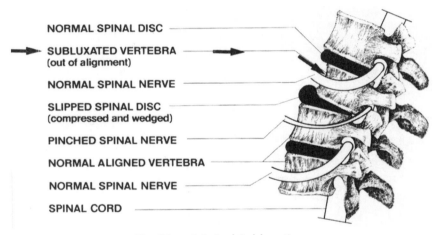

NORMAL SPINAL DISC

SUBLUXATED VERTEBRA
(out of alignment)

NORMAL SPINAL NERVE

SLIPPED SPINAL DISC
(compressed and wedged)

PINCHED SPINAL NERVE

NORMAL ALIGNED VERTEBRA

NORMAL SPINAL NERVE

SPINAL CORD

Fig. P6 — A Spinal Subluxation
Reprinted through the courtesy of Chiropractic Public Relations (CPR),
141 Blauvelt St. Teaneck, NJ 07666

In my opinion, this justifies the application of spinal manipulations (adjustments or stimulations) as an integral part of the healing process where leaky gut is involved. The chiropractor and the osteopath are the only health practitioners who are specifically trained in the technique of spinal manipulation; in fact it is the mainstay of their professions.

The areas of the spine designated are the 5th, 6th, and 7th thoracic (dorsal) vertebrae, located between the shoulder blades to be precise. This is the area where the spinal segments emit the nerves of the sympathetic chain that supply the entire upper intestinal tract. Emanating from these segments are the *afferent* (going out) and *efferent* (going in) nerves that supply the intestinal walls. To be in a healthy state, they must be flowing freely in both directions, or, a sort of short circuit takes place, which is often imperceptible for many years. The adjustments, and/or stimulations of these areas by the chiropractor or osteopath, can greatly influence the normal functioning of the alimentary canal, which of course includes the entire intestinal tract. As noted above, I personally center my efforts on the 5th through the 9th thoracic vertebrae, but also the 3rd cervical, and the 4th lumbar since they are the spinal segments that supply the primary nerve centers (ganglia) of the body.

The nerves that emit from the 5th through the 9th dorsals come together and form the celiac ganglion, sometimes referred to as the *abdominal brain* or solar plexus. It supplies the nerve channels to the heart, lungs, pancreas, spleen, kidneys, stomach, and small intestine (our focal point of investigation).

In reading 4000-1, Cayce attributes the basic cause of a person suffering from the skin condition psoriasis to *one* subluxation in the thoracic spine! The reason for such a dramatic declaration was also explained: As mentioned earlier, the spinal misalignment has an adverse influence on the blood circulatory system of the walls of the intestine, as well as organs of the entire viscera, and cause an "impoverishment" of the cellular structure of the organ(s) involved. If the misalignment is not corrected by manual or other means, the cells begin to break down for lack of proper nourishment, and thus the walls of the intestine gradually deteriorate. This may take time to develop and is often difficult to detect. X–rays or even MRIs may not reveal the insidious process, but nevertheless, it is taking place.

When this occurs, the patient's immune system is compromised. The patient becomes less able to ward off infection, allergies, foreign invaders (or what are *interpreted* as foreign invaders), etc. until at last the last organ supplied cries out for help—be it the skin, kidneys, heart, lungs, or brain!

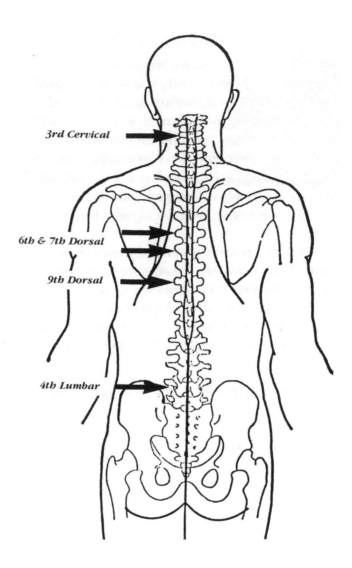

Fig. P7 — Primary Areas of the Spine to be Adjusted in LGS
Gray's Anatomy (26th ed. Philadelphia, Lea and Febiger, 1954. 30th Ed, Pub.
1985, Carmine D. Clemente, Ed.) Labeled by the author

A vicious cycle, but it is one that can often be reversed by correcting the basic cause. It is remarkable how quickly the body can recover once the basic cause is determined and corrected. I frequently recall something I learned in pathology class while still a student: *Allow one month of recovery time for every year the patient has been sick!* That's not a bad ratio, but of course, that assumes the basic cause of the problem has been recognized in the first place.

When Hippocrates (470–410 BC), the father or modern medicine, said, "Look well to the spine for the cause of disease," I would say the good doctor certainly knew whereof he spoke!

A Most Interesting Story—Polycythemia Vera, Diabetes, and Spinal Adjustments

When I hear of a substance, be it a drug, vitamin, mineral, compound or whatever, that is purported to cure everything from baldness to cancer, I look upon such exaggerated claims as a hallmark of charlatanism. This holds true, as far as I am concerned, with different schools of thought and therapies as well. Each in their own right may certainly benefit the patient, but to look upon any one concept as an answer to all man's ills borders on the ridiculous, and is and should be held suspect to a critical mind.

Nevertheless, I would be remiss if I did not at least report to my readers the true story of one of my patients who followed the LGS regimen and found extremely beneficial results from more than one illness he was faced with.

Mr. W.S. suffered from polycythemia vera, a condition in which the red blood cell mass is pathologically increased. The cause and cure are unknown. Medical management, however, was able to keep the problem relatively under control.

I relate this case with the permission of my patient, without attempting any scientific explanation as to physiologic processes that took place, which brought about a successful result. A few thoughts on the matter are briefly mentioned toward the end of the chapter which may be worthy of consideration. I simply report the situation, what we did, and the end result. My obligation is to report the truth. It remains the right of my readers to believe or disbelieve.

Polycythemia Vera

After delivering a lecture on psoriasis as it related to the Leaky Gut Syndrome at the Dag Hammarskjöld Library Auditorium at the United Nations in New York on October 29, 1980, I was met backstage by a distinguished gentleman, Mr. W.S., who was at the time president of the United Nations Parapsychology Society, which had sponsored the program. After a brief introduction, he informed me that he wished to visit my office and possibly become my patient. I assumed he had psoriasis and made an appointment. He arrived on schedule, and I began taking down his case history. If it was psoriasis, it was one of the strangest cases I had ever seen. His face was beet–red and the tips of his ears were as blue as ink. The rest of his body, however, was milk–white. It was as though he had gone to the beach, buried his body in the sand up to his neck, and exposed only his head to the sun.

He informed me that the problem he had been suffering from for forty years was not psoriasis, but polycythemia vera, a condition that could become quite grave. Red blood cells (RBCs) are formed primarily in the bone marrow of the skeletal system. Normal RBC values in the adult male range from 4.7 to 6.1 million cells per microliter, and for females the count is 4.2 to 5.4 million cells per microliter according to the online *MedlinePlus Medical Encyclopedia*. This count may vary a bit under certain physical or environmental conditions and still be regarded as normal. A patient with polycythemia vera may have a red blood count *three times* as high as the norm! Medical management typically consists of phlebotomy, i.e., removing a pint of excess blood weekly to reduce high blood viscosity. In the case of Mr. W.S., an abnormally high blood pressure (170/110), a pulse rate of 80, and profuse sweating added to his dilemma. The work load of his heart (WLH) was 14,000 (normal ranging from 8,000 to 10,000) which indicated the heart was working nearly 50 percent harder than it should. (The work load of the heart is determined by multiplying the systolic blood pressure by the pulse rate.)

Without hesitation I informed him that this was a medical condition with which I had no experience and the only connection I had had with the disease was between the pages of a textbook. He understood but said, "Something in your film got to me!" At the time it was not clear to me what part of the film had resonated with him, but later we were to find out.

During our initial visit I asked the classic questions: "Any accidents? Any allergies? Any constipation?" The answer was always, "No—nothing wrong there." Finding nothing particularly out of order, I agreed with him to run a trial series of treatments based on the leaky gut syndrome. I made no promises.

Two weeks passed with no change in my patient. Frustration began to set in. Why was he not responding? I decided to review the questions. "Any accidents or allergies?" "No." "Any constipation?" "No, I go regularly every four or five days!" The lights went on for me. "Wait a minute—I thought you told me you had no constipation problem?" He firmly answered, "I don't." "Do you consider evacuating once every four or five days 'normal'?" He answered, "Yes, I do. That is what my doctor told me many years ago. When I told him I only move my bowels every four or five days and that I was *always constipated*, he told me that in my case it was normal!" The patient did not question his doctor's judgment and lived with this absurd belief for fifty-six years! When I informed him that proper evacuation meant at least once or even twice or three times a day, he was astounded. Our regimen now focused on cleansing the colon, developing daily bowel movements, and having spinal adjustments.

In a couple of weeks, the response now shifted from no reaction to a slight ray of hope. He began to feel better generally, and signs of increased energy and vitality began to appear. He began to move his bowels twice a week, then three times, until finally he was able to move them daily or every other day. His head started to return to a normal color, as did the rest of his body. His blood pressure steadily dropped, reducing the work load of his heart, and most important, his blood count approached the normal range. By the time our series of treatments was over, his blood pressure was 120/80 (normal); there was no constipation to speak of; and a normal red blood cell count was established.

Mr. W.S. not only gave me permission to use his name at any of my lectures, but four years later he also appeared in person and addressed my audience at the Fort Lee Historic Park Museum in Fort Lee, N.J., on June 9, 1984, as a living testimony to a successful outcome.

Six years after Mr. W.S.'s condition cleared, I requested a follow–up account of his current state of health. Here, for the benefit of my readers, reproduced by permission, are pertinent excerpts of his response to me dated May 10,1986:

> After giving up hope of finding a cure for my skin problems which plagued me for a good part of my life, I came in contact with a medical doctor (name omitted) in January 1975.
>
> I explained to him my constant irritation and itching all over my body with outbreaks of poison ivy like eruptions all over my neck area and face. After an extensive series of blood tests and physical examinations, he came to the conclusion that I had "Diabetes Mellitus—Polycythemia Vera" (quoted from his official letter). His treatment, also quoted from his letter, was "removal of 10cc of patient's blood from arm, injection of 1cc benadryl."
>
> This treatment was given to me once a month with a daily application of cortisone to my face and neck area. I was then able to tolerate myself.
>
> He told me this was not a cure and I would have to do this for the rest of my life.
>
> As time passed the treatment was getting less and less effective, with my face turning a deep red color.
>
> The doctor passed away just before your lecture at the United Nations in 1980. I was then looking for another approach to a cure. Although his treatment was partially effective, it was not a cure.
>
> Your presentation at the United Nations was a godsend. It seemed you were describing all my ailments. The rest is history.
>
> As co-founder of the United Nations Parapsychology Society, it was my good fortune to co-sponsor your appearance at the U.N., not knowing it would affect my life.
>
> Immediately after my visit to your office, with the understanding that this was an experiment, I started the treatment. I cleansed my system with the apple diet and a series of high

colonics. Doing this, together with your diet and treatments, I was able in a couple of weeks to eliminate the cortisone application to my face and neck area. To this day my face is clear and of normal color without the use of cortisone.

Before your treatment I was 232 lbs. and on a low calorie diet. In following your diet I decided not to worry about calories so as not to interfere with the experiment. In spite of an increased calorie intake of at least 100%, my weight started to drop. The result was a loss of 30 pounds in three months.

If this treatment was given by the medical profession it would be a lifesaver for countless thousands of people.

I am pleased to be of help in your crusade to bring this treatment to the general public and will be available for any future project.

Best wishes,

W.S.

I have never had a case of polycythemia vera before or since Mr. W.S. Whether or not the regimen would work on other cases can only be answered by future experiences when and if they come. But here is one case in which it did indeed work.

The question to determine is what part of the therapy was the most beneficial. Was it the diet that had an effect on the leaky gut? Was it the cleansing of the bowel which allowed proper drainage of internal toxins? Was it the spinal adjustments, ensuring nerve supply to the intestinal wall? It could be, when one considers the findings of Schafer: "Removal of the paravertebral chain of sympathetic ganglia was followed by a gradual return of the erythrocyte (red blood cell) count to normal (in animals). A similar result followed paravertebral sympathectomy in a patient suffering from polycythemia." (Best and Taylor, 1955, p. 58)

At least Schafer proved there is a spinal connection with red blood cell formation, if nothing else. Spinal adjustments directly affect the spine, and, in turn physiologic function. It may have played more of a part in the case of W.S. than even I realized. Or maybe it was the combination of all these things, which is the theory I favor.

The point is that the natural approach to a leaky gut was utilized in a case of polycythemia vera and the result was positive. This should remind us again of the reading previously quoted (2002-1) in which Cayce informs us that diseases have changed little but their classifications, a great deal.

It Was in the Readings!

Years passed before I learned, much to my amazement, that Cayce did, in fact, have not only one but four readings on polycythemia vera! It never occurred to me that such a relatively rare disease would be contained in the material. Not until I received a complimentary copy of Reba Ann Karp's monumental undertaking *The Edgar Cayce Encyclopedia of Healing*, did I find an excellent account on polycythemia vera.

I proceeded to read the report with feelings of great enthusiasm mixed with apprehension. Would the information by Ms. Karp contradict what I had found to be effective in the case of W.S.? Had I neglected certain facets of therapy that Cayce may have suggested? Did I do something that was ill-advised in the readings yet achieve beneficial results? All these questions occupied my mind as I began to study the short but informative article.

When I finished reading the two pages devoted to polycythemia vera, I closed my eyes, laid back on my chaise lounge, and gave thanks! Every measure called for in the readings was utilized on Mr. W.S. and nothing was contradictory! The therapeutic procedures called for in psoriasis were almost exact in every detail to that required in the treatment of polycythemia vera. The diet was particularly stressed, and the cause, at least in the cases recorded, was cited as being due to poor assimilation (leaky gut?) and elimination, with spinal misalignment (subluxation) particularly in the mid-dorsals as a major area of concern because of abnormal nerve impulses to the pancreas!

In another case, a diet of fruit juices and water was suggested to replace the lost plasma and lower the red blood cell count. A typical diet was to include citrus fruit or cereal at breakfast, raw vegetables at lunch, cooked vegetables with fish, fowl, or lamb at dinner. Sugar and highly starchy foods were to be avoided—sound familiar?

As a chiropractor, I was particularly interested in the following paragraph taken directly form Mrs. Karp's article:

The one reporting beneficial results was that of case 674, an eleven-year-old boy who received one reading for the illness. According to Cayce, an injury to the dorsal area of the spine had produced a subluxation that caused the pancreas to become overactive. The liver subsequently became sluggish and the kidneys overactive, resulting in the high red blood cell count.

Beneficial results were noted after the boy followed the treatments for one month. (Karp, 1986, p. 369)

This paragraph dispelled all doubt in my mind as to the possible influence the spinal adjustments had in the case of W.S.

Let's go back for a moment and recall the diagnosis of Mr. W.S.'s condition as recorded in his medical doctor's communication to him. He diagnosed his patient as having "diabetes mellitus—polycythemia vera"—a combined health problem.

I find it most significant to note that the patient also had diabetes on top of his polycythemia and the organ primarily involved with diabetes is, as you may have guessed, the pancreas! I called on W.S. on May 26, 1986, and asked about the status of the underlying condition of diabetes mellitus. He informed me that both conditions were perfectly under control—"no problem!"—was his answer to me. When the polycythemia cleared up, so did the diabetes!

This case illustrates vividly that a broadening and expansion of present day concepts on healing such diseases must eventually take place. If it is true that spinal adjustments, dietary control, and proper elimination together heals polycythemia vera, then it will remain true forever. The laws of healing will not change to conform to humanity's concept. We must change our concept to conform to the laws of healing!

6

●—●—●—●—●—●—●

The Long Arm of LGS

What struck me more than anything else when I began my research on the leaky gut phenomenon was how far–reaching it
seems to be! There is no question in my mind that it is the *underlying*
cause of many, many diseases, especially the degenerative diseases. I
found scientific references that linked the leaky gut to disorders one
would not necessarily suspect of being related, such as obsessive–compulsive disorders (OCD), schizophrenia, mental depression, and other
psychochemical reactions. Other maladies of a different nature include:
rheumatoid arthritis, psoriatic arthritis, ankylosing spondylitis,
fibromyalgia, and similar musculo–skeletal disorders. In other words,
because the condition centers on the gastrointestinal area and digestion, as stated earlier, the effects of a damaged intestinal wall reach out
to other structures and systems far more widely than meets the eye.
These are referred to as *target organs.*

If a damaged intestinal wall, therefore, ultimately ends up by pollut-
ing the blood circulatory system, then the pollution is carried to wher-
ever the blood goes. And where does the blood go? Everywhere, to
every cell that constitutes the human body!

It Was in the Readings!

This concept of a leaky gut as being the origin of many, *seemingly* unrelated, diseases of the body was, in fact, addressed in the Edgar Cayce discourses themselves. In speaking of psoriasis and what toxic blood can do if it is not thrown off through the skin, consider 943-17:

> Would this not be thrown off in the epidermis [skin], or the lymph and capillary circulation, with this particular condition of this body, the intestinal tract would be full of pinholes; or, were it to go to the lungs, there would be tuberculosis; were it to go to the valves of the heart, there would be heart trouble—as would be called; were it to go to the liver, it would be cirrhosis of the liver; were it to go to the spleen, it would be a hardening of one end of it; were it to go to the brain, it would be [a] softening of the brain; were it to go to the glands of the throat or thyroids, it would be that of goiter; or were it to settle in some other portion—were it to *settle*—it would become a tumor of some character or nature.

Could it be any clearer? A reader may have his own beliefs as to the efficacy of The Edgar Cayce readings compared to scientific discoveries, but I believe one thing is certain: when the two agree with each other, it should be a clear sign to stand up and take notice.

The Far-Reaching Effects of LGS

If conditions such as psoriasis, psoriatic arthritis, and eczema, are due to a leaky gut, and the cause of the problem lies in the daily diet, why couldn't the cause of the following diseases also be due to a faulty diet primarily, as well as to poor eliminations over a long period of time?

According to Dr. Galland, there are many diseases associated with the Leaky Gut Syndrome. The following list is taken from his online article "Leaky Gut Syndromes: Breaking the Vicious Cycle."

Diseases Associated with Increased Intestinal Permeability
Inflammatory bowel disease
Infectious enterocolitis

Spondyloarthropathies
Acne
Eczema
Psoriasis
Urticaria
Cystic fibrosis
Pancreatic insufficiency
AIDS, HIV infection
Hepatic dysfunction
Irritable bowel syndrome with food intolerance
CFIDS
Chronic arthritis/pain treated with NSAIDS
Alcoholism
Neoplasia treated with cytotoxic drugs
Celiac disease
Dermatitis herpetiformis
Autism
Childhood hyperactivity
Environmental illness
Multiple food and chemical sensitivities
(Source: www.mdheal.org/leakygut.htm)

How LGS Affects Certain Conditions

Increased permeability of the intestinal mucosal barriers appears to correlate with a number of frequently seen clinical disorders. From the list given above, I have chosen to deal with a few of the diseases (some in greater detail, some in less) in the pages that follow.

Inflammatory Bowel Disease (IBD)

It has been consistently reported that increase in the permeability of the gut wall coincides with small bowel inflammation. As early as 1972 it was proposed that a break of the intestinal barrier is fundamental to the development of intestinal inflammation. Crohn's disease (an inflammation at the junction of the small intestine and the colon) has been shown to be more extensive than sometimes apparent using macroscopic approaches.

Concerning elimination diets, when patients with Crohn's disease were placed on an elemental diet, their permeability improved significantly, which coincided with marked clinical improvement. (Bell et al, 1999, p. G–30)

Inflammatory Joint Disease (IJD)

This includes the various forms of arthritis, of which there are at least 100 identified. The most common are Rheumatoid (RA) and Degenerative Joint Disease (DJD), Psoriatic arthritis (PA) and Ankylosing spondylitis, a condition in which the entire spine is affected, turning it into what is called "poker" spine by radiologists, and in which in advanced stages all flexibility of the spine comes to a complete halt. Studies have demonstrated that the above conditions include increased intestinal permeability, which may be an important factor to consider in the pathogenesis of these diseases.

A study was done to determine the influence of diet on arthritis, and the conclusion was that fasting leads to improvement of rheumatoid arthritis by reducing the permeability of the gut. Another study showed that spondyloarthropathies are triggered through the gut.

Having treated conditions of the spine for so many years, I have certainly had my fair share of spondyloarthropathies. Along with spinal manipulation (of a gentle nature), the best results were obtained with a change in diet, from highly acidic to highly alkaline, which is fostered throughout the Cayce readings. In addition to the change in diet and manipulation, the most gratifying results came about by the use of Cayce-recommended castor oil packs, combined with moist heat and massage. It is one of the most difficult conditions to treat, but with time and patience on the part of both patient and practitioner, beneficial results can be and have been attained. (There will be more on castor oil and its effective uses in Part II.)

Food Allergy

When it comes to the reaction of certain foods with different individuals, two things must be taken into consideration: Is it a food allergy or a food sensitivity? *Food allergy* is triggered by the immune system—a reaction that consistently occurs with the ingestion of *certain* foods, which cause functional changes in what is called "target organs." *Food sensitivity* refers to *all* adverse reactions to the ingestion of food.

"Andre, in a study of food allergy, concluded that 'the evaluation of intestinal permeability provides an objective means of diagnosing food allergy and assessing the effectiveness of anti-allergic agents.'" (Ball et al, 1999, p. G-30)

"Urticaria [hives] and atopic dermatitis [eczema] can be caused by the ingestion of certain foods. Andre showed that people with atopic dermatitis and those with urticaria demonstrated increased permeability when given an oral challenge of food that provoked symptoms." (Ball et al, 1999, p G-31)

Celiac Disease

The symptoms that characterize Celiac diseases are classic: indigestion, stomach bloating, chronic bouts between constipation and diarrhea, gas accumulation, skin eruptions, and in the case of children—a pendulous abdomen and failure to grow, a sure sign of maldigestion and malabsorption.

Just about every one of the above symptoms was present in one of my young patients, Z.A., whose story appears at the end of Part I. If ever there was an inspiring account with a successful conclusion, it is the story of young Z.A. The cause of his problem was due to *gluten intolerance*, which led to severe eczema.

Here again, the principle approach to healing this disease is first and foremost to avoid gluten–laden foods for about a week and watch the results. Other healing factors help the entire process, but the avoidance of the culprit, gluten, is paramount, because of the destructive effect it has on the gut wall of certain people. This is referred to as *gluten-sensitive enteropathy.*

In such a condition, permeability of large molecules may increase while permeability of small molecules decreases. Nutrients, if you remember, are small molecules. Therefore if they decrease in passing over into the blood stream, the cells become starved; normal absorption cannot take place. The decreased transcellular permeability to small, water-soluble molecules may lead to malnutrition; thus the reason for the lack of growth.

HIV Infection and AIDS (Human Immunodeficiency Virus and Acquired Immunodeficiency Syndrome)

Researchers are now looking at a link between intestinal permeability and HIV and AIDS. Tepper, in a recent study, looked at intestinal permeability in asymptomatic sick patients with HIV/AIDS, with and without diarrhea. This study indicates that patients with both AIDS and diarrhea have altered intestinal permeability, which would allow pathogens to cross over the mucosal barrier and invade the blood stream. Mannitol recovery decreased considerably in cases that tested positive for HIV. This suggests that as HIV progresses there is a loss of function in the inner wall of the intestines, bringing about a blockage of micronutrients from being absorbed. Malnutrition is the end result of such a condition, a characteristic of advanced stages of AIDS. (Ball et al, 1999, p. G-31)

Cystic Fibrosis

Cystic Fibrosis is caused by a gene defect identified in 1989. This tiny defect is a devastating one that affects many different glands in the body, including the pancreas, sweat glands, and glands of the digestive and respiratory system. (An extensive list of nutrients that may help cystic fibrosis may be found in *Prescription for Nutritional Healing*, by Dr. James and Phyllis Balch, pages 220–222.)

Intestinal permeability was studied recently with patients clearly defined as having Cystic Fibrosis or pancreatic insufficiency. In those studies, Lactulose, the larger molecule, penetrated the gut walls, compared to controls. The degree of gut wall permeability correlated with the level of duodenal trypsin and with the degree of undigested fat in the stool. As a suggestion, the authors recommended testing for urinary lactulose in that it may be useful in evaluating exocrine pancreatic function. (Author's Note: The Lactulose/Mannitol Challenge Test—Intestinal Permeability Assessment—is covered in Part II.)

Alcoholism

Alcoholics have elevated permeability. This is the conclusion reached by Bjarmason in his studies of alcoholic individuals. Even after two weeks of refraining from alcohol, the abnormality persisted. This increased permeability may account for problems that develop other than intestinal tissue damage. Bode reported that poisons derived from a damaged gut might play a role in liver disease. (Ball et al, 1999, p. G-32)

Aging

The people of the world, especially in the United States, are more conscious of the aging process than ever before. They spend thousands— yes, even millions—of dollars to look and feel young and to extend their lives to the outer limits. Cosmetics and anti-aging drugs constitute a multi-billion dollar industry; yet, how many people (including doctors!) think of looking to the gut for some answers? If they do, it is rare indeed.

An intriguing study on aging by Hollander concluded that "the intestinal barrier to the absorption of potentially harmful environmental substances may be less efficient in aging animals." (Ball et al, 1999, p. G-32)

Various studies show that aging rats have less ability to prevent larger size molecules from penetrating the intestinal mucosa. This can allow the antigenic or mutagenic compounds the ability to breech the gut barrier and to invade the bloodstream, which undoubtedly contributes to the breakdown of body cells. So, among other things, many researchers find a link between the gut interior and its effect upon the aging process. (Ball et al, 1999, p. G-32)

Edgar Cayce had much to say about the aging process. According to Cayce, our present lifespan should be anywhere from 121 to 150 years—

and we should be in good health! He attributes the relatively short lifespan, even though it has doubled since the beginning of the twentieth century, to our sedentary lifestyle, the consumption of too many processed foods, stress and anxiety, lack of fresh air and water, and to problems with the assimilation and absorption of even proper foods. And here is where we find a similarity with modern–day concepts of a leaky gut.

In the same way that science places emphasis on the intestinal villi and its role in LGS, Cayce brings our attention to the anatomical structures located in the lining of the small intestine known as "Peyer's Patches."

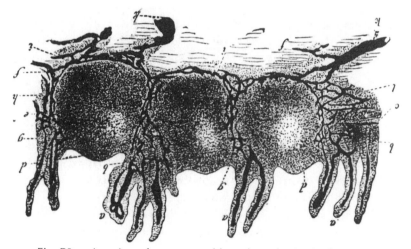

Fig. P8 — A series of aggregated lymph nodes in the lining
of the small intestine — Peyer's Patches
Gray's Anatomy (26th ed. Philadelphia, Lea and Febiger, 1954. 30th Ed.,
Pub. 1985, Carmine D. Clemente, Ed.)

Cayce considered these specialized lymph nodes as very important. These patches are abundant in the young, become indistinct in middle age, and can disappear completely in advanced years. The thymus gland is the master of the immune system, according to Dr. Harold J. Reilly in *The Edgar Cayce Handbook for Health Through Drugless Therapy*. He states also that "cells from the thymus migrate to other portions of the body (such as to the Peyer's Patches) and become centers of lymphatic activity." (Reilly and Brod, 1975)

Since the thymus gland is referred to as the "master of the immune system" and LGS is a major cause for the breakdown of the immune system, I would think that the Peyer's Patches Cayce speaks of deserve consideration as their deterioration in the aging process may give us a clue as to how we can thwart or delay the effects of old age.

Cayce goes further than that and suggests a remedy that may help regenerate these specialty glands located in the lining of the small intestine, which undoubtedly mingle among the intestinal villi or are at least in close proximity to them.

He recommends the *regular use of castor oil pack*—one of the most common remedies that I have used successfully through the years on many patients and on myself for various conditions. The wide use of this healing marvel is detailed in Dr. William McGarey's impressive account, *The Oil That Heals*.

The Anti-Aging Effect of Olive Oil

Olive oil has been considered one of the most beneficial oils ever consumed by the human species. It is one of the most digestible of all fats. Olive oil contributes to longevity by reducing the wear and tear of aging on body tissues, organs, and brain. It reduces the risk of heart disease and cancer and can protect against stomach ulcers.

It is not a good idea to cook with olive oil. Rather, grape seed oil or Canola oil should be used for cooking as high heat does not have the same breakdown effect on grape seed oil as it does on olive oil. After food is cooked, olive oil can be added for taste and nutritional value.

Much can be said about the healthfulness of olive oil and its beneficial effects upon the digestive tract. For one thing, olive oil combined with fresh garlic is a powerful countermeasure to the build-up of yeast within the intestinal mucosa, whereby it helps to prevent and destroy candida (yeast overgrowth).

Two Italian researchers, Viola and Mirella, suggested that olive oil relieved gastrointestinal disorders because it helped the natural rhythm of digestion. It reduces excess bile and free radicals while stimulating the pancreas. They further stated that "Owing to its balanced composition, olive oil has a protective effect upon the arteries, the stomach and the liver, it promotes growth during childhood and extends life expect-ancy." (Shaw)

Jerry Shaw quotes Andrew Weil, M.D., popular author of several books on natural healing, who has only good things to say about olive oil. Dr. Weil says that olive oil is the best and safest of all edible fats. "Replacing saturated fats in the diet with olive oil leads to a reduction of bad cholesterol (whereas, replacement with polyunsaturated vegetable oils lowers good cholesterol as well . . .)" says Weil, (Shaw)

Olive oil, a monounsaturate, has high amounts of oleic acid, which helps reduce the blood platelet clotting that can lead to heart failure. "Old age brings with it reduced digestive capacity and poor absorption of nutrients especially of vitamins and mineral salts." (Shaw) (Author's note: possibly due to the slow deterioration of the previously men-tioned Peyer's Patches.)

Olive oil has the best characteristics for digestibility and absorption, and acts as a mild laxative. Olive oil in its raw state is most beneficial. So here we have an age-old item that has been considered one of the most powerful anti-aging products since the days of Hippocrates be-cause of its nutritive value on the digestive system and all the structures thereof—olive oil! In my opinion, it will add life to your years and years to your life.

Vision

With so many conditions that the flesh is heir to, is it any wonder that the delicate membranes and structures of the eye do not escape the destructive effects of polluted blood? Not according to Robert Abel, Jr., M.D., author of *The Eye Care Revolution*. In Dr. Abel's view, the Leaky Gut Syndrome is something to be guarded against because it can affect vi-sion.

According to Dr. Abel, "Some of the same dietary deficiencies that contribute to leaking blood vessels are also associated with leaky gut syndrome or intestinal permeability defects. Once the lining of the gas-trointestinal system is damaged, food is not properly digested; instead, it ferments in the colon, causing gas and pain. Leaky gut syndrome appears to contribute to the development of autoimmune disorders like inflammatory bowel disease, rheumatoid arthritis and lupus, food and chemical sensitivities and bacterial infections (septicemia)." (Abel, 1999, p. 165) Dr. Abel continues, "Poor digestion results in starvation of the eye and the rest of the body over many years before the joints ache, the heart skips a beat, and the small print looks wavy."

Dr. Abel lists the following supplements which he believes can be helpful in healing a leaky gut:

- Glutamine, a deficiency of which results in intestinal damage
- Gamma linolenic acid (GLA), an amino acid that acts as an anti-inflammatory agent
- Acidophilus, the "good" bacteria
- Vitamin A, which supports the intestinal lining
- N–acetyl–D–glucosamine (NAG), which promotes the formation of a healthy gut lining
- Phosphatidylcholine, which protects the gastrointestinal lining from chemicals
- Gamma–oryzanol, an extract of rice bran oil that is a potent anti-oxidant (Abel, 1999)

Dr. Abel's Tip:
The macula has a powdery yellow pigment that absorbs dangerous blue light on UV wavelengths. This fat–soluble pigment is rebuilt by lutein and zeaxanthin, found in green leafy vegetables, eggs, and corn; so eat plenty of these foods.

"Macular degeneration is a disease of starvation, especially of the good fats (like DHA and the other Omega–3 fats). Fat–soluble vitamins and enzymes, working with the good fats, protect against the constant free–radical formation caused by sunlight. Improve your digestion and increase the Omega–3 essential fatty acids in your diet." (Abel, 1999, p. 165)

In speaking of the role digestion plays relative to the eye, Dr. Abel is quite direct: "A reduced amount of stomach acid can lead to poor diges-tion, as can an imbalance of the good intestinal flora and too many toxins in the colon. Antibiotics are notorious for upsetting this balance." (Abel, 1999)

He goes on to say that a deficiency of stomach acids results in less absorption of many essential nutrients which can result in lack of anti-oxidants and reduced ability to fight free-radical damage in the eye. He states that "what's good for the digestion is good for the eye. Remember, it takes only twenty minutes for the nutrients (or toxins) you eat to reach your eye, and certain eye diseases correlate with dietary deficiency. Macular degeneration is a disease of poor digestion."

Dr. Abel also makes reference to the fact that aloe vera, licorice root, comfrey root, ginger and garlic all have anti-inflammatory effects on the gut. He further advises: "Be good to your gastric mucosa. A healthy intestinal lining protects against the development of leaky gut syndrome, which can cause inflammatory bowel disease and other autoimmune disorders." (Abel, 1999, p. 284)

Multiple Sclerosis (MS)—Possibly Linked to LGS?

During my internship at the Chiropractic Hospital in Denver, I worked on thirty to forty patients per day, six days a week. All manner of ailments came to the hospital for chiropractic adjustments, massage therapy, rehabilitation, and any other technique that fell within our scope of practice. I was surprised to see several multiple sclerosis (MS) patients as part of our daily routine.

The cause of multiple sclerosis was unknown then as it still is now. The textbooks tell us what happens in the brain cells, but why it happens still eludes the researchers. Many theories as to its cause have been proposed over the years, i.e., infection, intoxication, nutritional deficiency, even thrombo phlebitis. Still a mystery, the disease continues to occur more frequently.

Not until I entered private practice after my internship did I take the works of Edgar Cayce seriously. Here, for the first time, I found a possible answer to this enigma, as I later found for so many other diseases.

Of the sixty-nine MS patients Cayce gave discourses for, forty were said to have MS due to a *lack of gold* in the system (reading 907-1). Now the only way a patient can suffer from a lack of gold in the system is that there is not enough of it in the diet—or—*what there is in the diet is not absorbed.* In his discourse on multiple sclerosis in the *Physician's Reference Notebook* published by the A.R.E. Press, Walter N. Pahnke, M.D., says,

"[The reason for the lack of gold] was tied to a defect in the assimilating system (by this was probably meant the digestive system) which in turn was kept in proper balance from the glands. Because the glands were in turn dependent upon the proper amount of gold in the system, this would apparently lead to a circular feedback relationship between gold, the glands, and the assimilating system." (Physicians Reference Notebook, 1968, p. 152)

Cayce provided us with a whole array of therapeutic suggestions—everything from the wet cell appliance, massage, spinal adjustments, diet, and others. Gold chloride, however, was by far the most frequent recommendation (using the wet cell appliance—which is a study in itself). These measures were suggested *after* the condition of MS was established in the body. The question here, however, is whether or not MS could be prevented or later helped by taking into account the effect that LGS may have had on the condition.

According to Dr. H.J. Reilly, the foods that contain adequate amounts of gold are: carrots, salsify (oyster plant), and shellfish. In other words, it is not a mineral that is hard to come by. I favor the second theory—that what gold there is in the diet, for one reason or another, is not absorbed and transferred to the body cells.

Just a Thought:

Remember the *protein carriers* we spoke of in an earlier chapter? It is a physiological fact that minerals such as gold, copper, zinc, and others, although minuscule, are vital to the functioning organism. In order for them to reach the body cells, however, they must "hitch-on" to a protein carrier in order to cross over the intestinal barrier supplied by the gut lumen. It was also brought out that if the gut wall is compromised by inflammation, injury, allergens, parasites, etc., it cannot perform its function as a carrier of metals across the barrier. It very well could be that gold, being a metal, may fall into this category.

Whenever we think of gold, we automatically think of its monetary value and leave it at that. Who ever thinks of this metal as vital to health? Unless you are a nutrition-minded individual (doctor or patient) it will pass unnoticed. Now, with the ever-growing interest in proper nutrition, perhaps this theory will at least be investigated. Cayce gives us a clue as to how to proceed. The question is: Who, in the right position, will pick up on it and take it seriously?

From a pathological point of view, MS shows multiple patches of degeneration which appear to occur in the white matter of the brain and spinal cord, rather than the gray. The lesions may appear as small as a pinhead to more than a centimeter in diameter.

It is the axon sheath (covering) that demyalizes, eventually leading to the breakdown and disappearance of the axon itself, leaving scar tissue, and thereby having its dysfunctioning effect on the neurological impulses. (Chusid and McDonald, 1954, p. 247)

All manner of treatments have been investigated and tried, usually with disappointing results: fever therapy, antibiotic therapy, protein shock, drugs of one kind and another, as well as bee stings—that many people claim helped when all else failed. The taking of granular lecithin has also been advocated to help regenerate the myelin sheath, and in at least one case of mine, it seemed to have been beneficial. Since there was no follow-up, however, this cannot be considered impressive.

Autism

Ten years ago, few people had ever heard the word *autism*, but today it is recognized as a growing problem all across America and elsewhere. Three to six children of every thousand have autism and boys are four times more likely to have it than girls, according to the U.S. National Institute of Neurological Disorders and Stroke.

Autism is a condition affecting children primarily from the toddler age into their twenties. Symptoms include a refusal or inability to speak; inability to control one's body, wherein the individual may throw up the hands suddenly or stare into space or at some inconsequential object; failure to appropriately engage with others socially; lack of interest in self-care and hygiene; or a tendency to violence, as in the case of a young girl who in one day broke every window in her house and punched holes in the walls.

On the Web site www.candidafree.net, Mark and Alyson Cobb include a quote from a Dr. Glen Gibson, of the University of Reading, Berkshire, England, who notes regarding autism that "Other symptoms may be hyperactivity, loss of eye contact, decreased vocalization (i.e., loss of language), poor academic and other similar social deficits. Other similar disorders exist. These include Asperger Syndrome (AS), Attention Deficit Hyperactivity Disorder (ADHD), Persuasive Developmental Disorder (PDD), and many others, where symptoms are similar to autism but specific differences are demonstrated."

In September and October of 2006, the *Record* newspaper of Bergen County, New Jersey, carried a six-part special report titled "In Autism's Grip." According to the *Record* report: "The number of children in New Jersey afflicted with autism has multiplied more than 30 times in the last 14 years: from 234 in 1991 to 7,400 in 2005, according to the Department of Education. The rising numbers may be evidence of an epidemic. Autism touches everyone. It creates headaches for parents and commands millions in tax dollars. But still there is no cure."

Researchers at the Center for Advanced Biotechnology and Medicine, a joint institute of Rutgers University and the University of Medicine and Dentistry of New Jersey (UMDNJ) are studying a possible genetic defect in the condition and the brain chemistry involved. Many other research centers throughout the country have launched similar studies hoping to find the root cause of the condition.

In the second of the *Record* series on autism, Dr. Julia Bramwell, a pediatrician who runs the Parsippany office of the New Jersey Hyperebaric Oxygen Therapy Office, is quoted as saying "One of the many theories is that autism is an autoimmune problem that causes inflammation of the nervous system or the gut, so this (oxygen therapy) is one way to decrease the inflammation." (Washburn, 2006) What strikes me as profound is that they referred to *inflammation of the gut* as having a possible link to the condition.

In an Internet article by Max Bingham, "Autism and the Human Gut Flora," he references Dr. Glen Gibson, who believes that there is a possible link between autism and the human gut flora. Dr. Gibson also explains that research in this area is sparse because of the unwillingness of the orthodox medical establishment to adopt treatments suggested by previous research into autism.

It appears, according to Dr. Gibson, that yeast (candida in particular), as well as clostridia, may play an important role in the development of autism. He suggests that the control of the growth of these species may reduce the severity of autism but is unlikely to offer a cure. The fact is, however, that this approach, dietary control, has never been truly researched since the orthodox medical establishment views this approach as "irrelevant." (It never fails to amaze me how such a conclusion can be reached when serious scientific research regarding a dietary approach to this disease has never been undertaken.)

So, the limited research has its drawbacks. Nevertheless, until true scientifically constructed testing is done, this is all we have to go on. Personally, I think it is relevant and should be looked upon with an open mind.

The following is taken directly from the article by Max Bingham, quoting Dr. Gibson's findings:

1. Following treatment with antifungal drugs and gluten and casein free diet, a child rated as having severe autism improved to such an extent that the child was classed as a higher functioning individual with autism.

2. It has been shown that children with autistic symptoms, after being tested for urinary metabolites, had extremely high values of *tartaric acid*. The only source of tartaric acid is *yeast*.

3. Many reports have suggested that autistic symptoms often occur after the child has been treated for otitis media (ear infections). It is common to treat otitis media with broad spectrum antibiotics. Intestinal overgrowth of yeast and certain anaerobic bacteria are a well documented outcome of the administration of broad spectrum antibiotics. (Kennedy and Volz, 1983; Danna et all, 1991; Ostfield et al, 1977; Kinsman et al, 1989; Van der Waaij, 1987; Samsonic et al, 1993, 1994b.) It is not clear however, why other children take large amounts of antibiotics for one reason or another but do not develop autism.

4. It is estimated that a large percentage of autistic children have a significant immune dysfunction.

5. It is not uncommon to find that children with autism experience improved symptoms following removal of gluten and casein from the diet.

6. Clostridium tetani is a ubiquitous anaerobic bacillus that is

known to produce a potent neurotoxin. Once in the brain, the tetanus neurotoxin disrupts the release of neurotransmitters. This may explain the wide variety of behavioural deficits apparent in autism.

7. It has been shown that incompletely broken down portions of gluten and casein may be crossing the gut into the blood and having an opioid effect in autistic children. (Bingham, n.d.)

So, the bottom line in Dr. Gibson's account is that: *While it will not cure this disorder (autism) modifications of gut flora function might improve symptoms significantly.*

Johnson & Johnson won U.S. approval to market Risperdal (its best selling drug for schizophrenia) for autism symptoms in children ages five to sixteen. It can be prescribed for children who demonstrate signs of aggression, temper tantrums, deliberate self-injury, and rapid mood swings, according to the Food and Drug Administration (FDA) on October 6, 2006.

The most common side effects of Risperdal include drowsiness, constipation, fatigue, and weight gain, said the FDA. Risperdal relieved aggression by more than 50 percent in a study published in the August 1, 2002, edition of the *New England Journal of Medicine*. The drug, however, helped children who harm themselves, as well as those with symptoms such as temper tantrums, agitation, unstable moods, and aggression. The drug didn't treat the autism itself, only the symptoms. (Rapaport and Cortez, 2006)

What would I do if I were faced with the problem of autism? I would certainly treat it as an offshoot of the Leaky Gut. I would take my patient off all refined sugar or sugar in any form. I would incorporate the gluten-free diet and keep them off oats, wheat, rye, and barley. No junk food would be allowed, as well as anything that would feed yeast. I would at the least recommend an intake of plenty of water and place the patient on a low acid/high alkaline diet. Then I would wait and observe carefully, looking for small signs of improvement. They might be tiny signs at first—but it is moving in the right direction, not the speed of improvement, that would be significant. As always, time and patience would be the keys, in addition to the dietary changes!

There May Be Another Way

William Crook, M.D., has a section in his book *The Yeast Connection Handbook* that zeroes in on autism and adds light to the subject of LGS. He covers many aspects of the disorder from a different perspective and offers eight recommendations in dealing with autism. Of particular interest to me was the eighth: "After the course of antibiotics has been completed, I recommend continuing the Nystatin and probiotics, two or three times daily for several weeks. Here's why: Nystatin discourages the growth of yeast in the intestinal tract and the probiotics replace friendly bacteria. These products help heal the 'leaky gut,' lessen the absorption of milk, wheat, and other allergens and decrease the chances of your child developing repeated ear problems." (Crook, 2000, pp. 89–90)

For years the researchers have tried to discover a drug for autism at the cost of millions upon millions of dollars and have concluded: "No drugs are approved in the U.S. for calming children with autism, and their behavior can make it difficult for them to benefit from education and therapeutic programs . . . " (Washburn 2006, p. A14)

Has it ever occurred to the researchers to try a change in diet? Or would that just be too simple?

A Story Worth Telling

To my readers who may still not be convinced that poor diet or overuse of antibiotics play a significant role in cases of autism and/or ADHD (Attention Deficit Hyperactivity disorder), I offer the following e-mail I received on November 13, 2007.

> Dr. Pagano,
> I wanted to share my story about my son S.D. At the age of four he was diagnosed with ADHD and some autistic spectrum symptoms. His symptoms included irritability, hyper-activity, anger, poor social skills, hand flapping, inability to follow directions, inappropriate behaviors and severe mood swings. He was in four different preschools, as each stated that they did not have the staff to handle such a boy.
> I went to my pediatrician and was given a prescription. I

decided at that time there had to be another way. I read and searched the Internet and spoke with many, many alternative doctors. There was one common theme that I found to be helping: diet. I threw out all the treatments my son was given, all the medicines, mega-doses of vitamins and injections and concentrated on diet.

What S.D. needed was a diet that corrected his years of antibiotic use and poor diet. He began eating fruits, vegetables, good protein and yogurt. It was a very basic, but healthy, plan. Slowly, I saw a change. He was not able to color in the lines at the age of five—and now at age eight he dreams of being an artist and creates impressive drawings and has the neatest writing of anyone in his class. He went from having no confidence and no friends, to a very confident boy with a healthy social life. His teachers used to call me almost every day with some problem, and today there are no calls and excellent reports.

Today, since his "gut" is repaired he is able to eat almost anything. However, if he does overdo it on a certain food, we begin to see some symptoms again. We do not fear that though because we know he can get right back on track and the symptoms simply disappear.

There are a few doctors who understand this natural approach to repair the gut and I am glad Dr. Pagano that you are one of them! Edgar Cayce told us the answer many years ago, we just need to listen

L.D. (Permission granted for reproduction.)

Initials used only in keeping with the patient's right to privacy.

I had the pleasure of meeting young S.D. personally on November 9, 2007. Rarely have I met an eight–year–old with such keen perception and intelligence. I asked him what he thought played a part in his previous difficulty. His answer was sharp and direct: "When I ate chocolate bars and Tootsie Rolls, I went cuckoo!"

Scleroderma

Scleroderma (hard skin) is a condition where "the body turns to stone," as it is often described. It is really a systemic condition that involves collagenous connective tissue, but the skin is the most visible organ in which the hardening of such is observed. All the internal organs can be involved: the kidneys, lungs, heart, liver, and even the arteries and glands

Scleroderma was one of the most devastating skin diseases that I encountered as a young intern in Denver. The afflicted patient was a woman who was in the last stages of her life when I met her. While there was nothing I nor anyone else could do to help her, many years later I had three separate cases of scleroderma come into my office in one year. Two of them responded, one did not—but she was already at the point of irreversibility when she first came to me. She had been under medical care for several years before I first saw her, but try as the doctors might, it was just too late.

The second case, however, a woman whom I will call Cathy, was different. After being under extended medical care, she found her way to my office in the hope of trying a more natural approach. For this I turned exclusively to the Edgar Cayce material. In his works he emphasized that scleroderma was primarily due to a malfunction of the glands of the body, principally the thyroid, adrenal, and liver. With the hormones of these glands malfunctioning, a tubercle bacillus or germ in the lymphatics of the skin itself occurs. The glandular deficiency creates a *lack of nutrition* in the circulation of the skin itself which affects the lymph flow. I followed the same procedure suggested for psoriasis, eczema, and psoriatic arthritis with two extra inclusions: a *charred oak keg* and castor oil. All other measures—the high–alkaline diet, olive oil/peanut oil massages, colonic irrigations, etc.—were followed.

The charred oak keg was employed since the woman had scleroderma with lung involvement. There was crystallization of the lung taking place. The charred oak keg is exactly what it implies: an oak keg that has been charred on the inside. To this was added 100 proof Apple Brandy that filled the bottom half of the keg. A breathing tube was supplied and inserted in the center of the keg that allowed the patient to breathe the fumes generated in the upper half of the keg. This procedure was advised for many problems of the respiratory system: asthma, emphysema, tuberculosis, pneumonia, and other such problems. The protocol was successful as is evidenced by her letter to me dated March 8, 1992:

Dear Dr. Pagano,
I'm writing you this letter to inform you of the results of my
tests I had run at Lahey Clinic. I went to Lahey on February 4,
5, 6. They did a pulmonary test which measured the amount
of air I take into my lungs and checked my blood gases. I'm
pleased to tell you the test turned out great. My lungs have
improved from last year. I have 97% oxygen in my blood. The
doctors couldn't believe it. They said that they have never
seen that before. When you have a thickening of the lung as I
did, it does not improve; it can stay the same but it will not
improve. Well, Doc, we proved them wrong—and I'm living
proof it can happen. I wish you could have been there to see
how confused they were because they couldn't explain it—it
was great! I know what did it though. I feel using the charred
oak keg and following the diet you gave me and following the
Cayce readings has made a major change in my health. I want
to thank you for everything you have done for me.
Sincerely,
Cathy

What, you may ask, does a charred oak keg have to do with the
Leaky Gut Syndrome? Let's remember that the leaky gut causes *systemic*
problems, the list of which can be staggering. Scleroderma is a systemic
condition; therefore, it must be treated systemically if results are to be
realized. In Cathy's case, her lungs became affected by the scleroderma
and produced pulmonary complications. Clearing the lungs with the
charred oak keg gave her a higher oxygen capacity. This gave her immune system a boost and helped her build up her entire system. In the
meantime, the dietary changes from acid to alkaline which she incorporated helped the overall picture.

Arthritis

As mentioned earlier, there are about 100 forms of arthritis from
which people suffer. These are broken down into groups. There are those
listed as infectious, juvenile, gouty, traumatic, trophic, degenerative, inflammatory, and others. The group we are most concerned with here is
inflammatory arthritis, of which there are four types:
1. Psoriatic arthritis

2. Reiter's Syndrome
3. Ankylosing Spondylitis
4. Arthritis of Inflammatory Bowel Disease

All of the above have a genetic factor in common that renders the patient as having a predisposition to the disease. This does not, however, mean that a person whose family has a history of the tendency of the disease will necessarily get it. Nor does it answer why one person in a family will get it while others do not.

From the *Genova Diagnostic Laboratory Functional Assessment Resource Manual*, we find that increased permeability of the gut wall is seen in Rheumatoid Arthritis (the form closest to psoriatic arthritis), Reiter's Syndrome, Ankylosing Spondylitis, and Arthritis of Inflammatory Bowel Disease (IBD). Three, possibly four, of the different forms of inflammatory arthritis appear to have a leaky gut at the root of the problem.

Each of the above forms of arthritis is medically treated with aspirin and/or corticosteroids. There are always new drugs coming onto the market, all of which have side effects which are sometimes worse than the condition itself. Note that aspirin, corticosteroids, and other more powerful pharmaceuticals can have a destructive influence on the intestinal wall—the very thing that we are trying to avoid in regard to the leaky gut. That's why those pharmaceuticals are listed as the number one cause of mucosal breakdown.

Since we have reason to believe that there is a leaky gut involvement here, it seems logical to center our efforts on healing the leaky gut—which will, in time, theoretically, help solve the inflammatory process going on in these diseases.

From the standpoint of treating arthritis in general, the following may well apply equally to all four arthritic reactions:

1. Alkalize the system (primarily through diet).
2. Prevent any constipation.
3. Make pure water the primary liquid consumed.
4. Have more green leafy vegetables than any other food.
5. Take peanut oil (cold pressed) massages or baths with cold pressed peanut oil.
6. Use warm or hot castor oil packs, especially along the spine in cases of psoriatic arthritis and ankylosing spondylitis.

7. Refrain from all use of sugar and processed foods made with sugar.

8. Avoid all fried foods.

9. Exercise—by walking, swimming, cycling, etc. No contact sports.

10. Avoid the Nightshades: tomatoes, tobacco, eggplant, white potatoes, peppers, and paprika.

11. Include raw garlic, olive oil, and lemon in cases of yeast infection.

12. Avoid gluten products in cases of celiac disease.

And last but not least: *See yourself getting well—not worse!*

Results in Psoriatic Arthritis (PA)—It Really Works!

All I can offer my readers are written affidavits in the form of letters
and e–mails that I received from sufferers of various problems and the
results that those individuals obtained.

For instance, the following is a letter from a person suffering from
psoriatic arthritis that I received in the spring of 2006:

Dear Dr. Pagano,
I am from the Philippines and I came to America in March of
2001. Then I had the chance to attend the Worldwide Conference on Psoriasis in San Francisco of the same year. My condition then was really severe, with psoriatic arthritis and lesions
all over my body. I started reading your book as soon as I
came back to Los Angeles and could not put it down. Then I
ordered the cookbook a few weeks later.

I have been clear for more than 3 years now and even
though I am writing you only now, I would say it's never too
late because I know that I will be clear forever from now on.
Thank you very much for your research and dedication in trying to find a cure for psoriasis. Like most of your patients, I
have also gone to many doctors and found only temporary
relief. When my dermatologist from the Philippines, who told
me before that diet had nothing to do with my condition, saw
me clear and wearing short pants, she asked for your book
and said she will recommend it to her patients too.

When I first read your book, I had some questions and then
I got to the part where to order the herbal teas, so I called the
800 number listed at the back and lo and behold, it was you
who answered the phone. You were so kind and encouraging

and you stayed on for maybe 10 minutes or so, which was so
generous of you. That day I resolved to really make it work
and it did!

Once again, thank you very much and rest assured, in my
own little way, I will always try to educate people based on
the knowledge I got from your book about psoriasis and personally reach out to other patients and encourage them to
choose the natural healing alternative.

God bless and more power to you!

Very truly yours,

"Christine"

P.S. I got married last year and when I was in severe condition
in 2001, I thought nobody will ever want to marry me. I met
my husband then and he was my biggest supporter and encouraged me to follow and stick to the regimen. Thanks again
Dr. Pagano.

What is remarkable about the above letter is that I never met the
patient. She attended the address I gave at the 2001 World Conference
on Psoriasis, sponsored by the National Psoriasis Foundation (NPF). After buying my book, *Healing Psoriasis: The Natural Alternative*, she faithfully
followed the suggestions and actually did more to help herself than
anyone else. This should offer hope to others suffering with psoriatic
arthritis.

Pityriasis Rubra Pilaris (PRP)

Pityriasis Rubra Pilaris (PRP) is a disease of the skin that I have never
dealt with; yet, on October 14, 2002, I received an e-mail from a family
conveying their joy and excitement after results were obtained on the
husband when he followed my suggestions on healing a leaky gut. Their
letter is reproduced here:

Hi Dr. Pagano,

I contacted you a little over a year ago about my husband
who was diagnosed with Pityriasis Rubra Pilaris (PRP). At that
time, we lived in Minnesota and since have moved to Florida.
You told me that you believed your diet would work for him.

Well, I would like to *thank you* from the bottom of my heart. It has definitely cleared him. He has been on the diet on and off for over the past year, and in between things he tried acupuncture (at that time he did not follow your diet), and his skin got bad again. He then went back on the diet and he started clearing again. Our chiropractor supported us along the way. I must say we got no support from the dermatologist or family doctor.

At this time, he only has a little of the PRP on his body. It is on his upper back and lower arms and a little on his hands. (It doesn't itch and looks more like a discoloring of the skin.) He only oils his body once a day, he no longer has chills, he no longer has joint pain, the soles of his feet are back to normal and his thickened nails are returning to normal. I have before and after pictures if you are interested in looking at them . . .

. . . We believe so much in your approach, and we believe that if people would just be a little more open they could be helped also . . . Once again, thank you so much.
Sincerely,
M.H.

Incredibly, just two weeks later, on October 30, 2002, I was amazed to receive another e-mail from a different person regarding positive results obtained with the same disease!

Hello Dr. Pagano,
First let me say thank you so much for your research and work. I have been diagnosed in April 2002 with PRP and my liver could not handle the Accutane I was put on. I was taken off the Accutane the end of July and started your diet August 1. I saw dramatic results in 3 weeks. Now at the end of October I can claim to be pretty much clear from the PRP. I was very sick and 100% of my body was covered, red, peeling, itching and painful. I thank you so much for your work, you literally gave me my life back.

I was so sick and I do not ever want to go back there again. I value your opinion and advice . . . Thanks so much for everything; I could never thank you enough.
C.G.

Here we have examples of the reactions of thee different people. Although the diagnosis was two distinct skin problems, each responded to the regimen outlined for cases of Leaky Gut Syndrome. Most significant, in my opinion, is the last line of M.H.'s letter where she writes " .. . if people would be a little more open they could be helped also ... " How true—I couldn't have said it better myself!

7

———•——•——•——•——•——

Celiac Disease

I open this chapter on celiac disease with a quote taken directly from the Internet (as cited), since it seems to me to be the perfect introduction to the material that follows.

> Celiac disease is a digestive disease that damages the small intestine and interferes with absorption of nutrients from food. People who have celiac disease cannot tolerate the protein called *gluten*, found in wheat, rye, and barley. Gluten is found mainly in foods, but is also found in products we use every day, such as stamp and envelope adhesive, medicines, and vitamins.
>
> When people with celiac disease eat foods or use products containing gluten, their immune system responds by damaging the small intestine. The tiny, fingerlike protrusions lining the small intestine are damaged or destroyed. Called villi, they normally allow nutrients from food to be absorbed into the bloodstream. Without healthy villi, a person becomes malnourished, regardless of the quantity of food eaten. Because the body's own immune system causes the damage, celiac disease is considered an *autoimmune disorder*. However, it is also

classified as a disease of malabsorption because nutrients are not absorbed. Celiac disease is also known as celiac sprue, nontropical sprue, and gluten-sensitive enteropathy.
Celiac disease is a genetic disease, meaning it runs in families. Sometimes the disease is triggered—or becomes active for the first time—after surgery, pregnancy, childbirth, viral infection, or severe emotional stress. (NDDIC Web site, n.d.)

Gluten Intolerance

Gluten Intolerance is also a fancy way of saying that a person's body can't handle gluten. So, what is gluten? You ingest it any time you have a slice of bread or a bowl of cereal (unless it is gluten-free). So, what does that have to do with LGS? Gluten is one of the recognized irritants of the gut wall, especially in people who are gluten intolerant. *The Leaky Gut Syndrome can be caused by anything that damages the gut wall.* Gluten is most assuredly one of those damaging factors.

Gluten is a mixture of protein fragments found in common cereal grains. Wheat is the only grain considered to contain true gluten (this includes semolina, durum, spelt, triticale, and kamut). Other grains such as rye and barley also contain similar protein fragments that can cause problems for those who have intolerance to gluten.

Gluten intolerance has been recognized for nearly 2,000 years in Greece. In India, intestinal diseases, including what we consider to be celiac sprue and other celiac diseases were described in medical literature, written in Sanskrit, as early as 1,500 B.C. In modern times, celiac disease is designated as a childhood disease, whereas in adults it is referred to as celiac sprue or non–tropical sprue.

In the publication *Gluten Intolerance* by Beatrice Trum Hunter, we learn that, although the cause of the disease is still in question, it could be due to lack of enzymes, an inborn metabolic error, or, shall we say, "genetic" in nature. Hunter explains: "This lack of enzymes leads to an incomplete breakdown of gluten protein and the accumulation in the gastrointestinal lumen (gut wall) of toxic peptides (undigested proteins) from a gluten protein. Normally, as in people without a gluten intolerance problem, the enzyme would break down and detoxify gluten before it could damage intestinal villi [Preventing a leaky gut?]." (Hunter, 1987)

Another theory is that it may be due to an immunologic defect which may inactivate many of the gastrointestinal epithelial cells. These epithelial cells line the inner lumen (wall) of the intestines. In other words, Hunter gives us reason to suspect gluten as being damaging to the walls of the intestines, which ultimately have a part in producing LGS. Most people, of course, can handle gluten without a problem. But, for those who can't, the only known treatment is to *avoid gluten in any form*.

Increasingly there are products available that can be used as a substitute for wheat and other gluten–containing products. *Kasha*, which is wheat– and gluten–free, makes a wonderful alternative to rice or potatoes with a cooked meal, or it can even be used as a breakfast cereal. Kasha has long been popular in Europe and is now becoming more known in the US. Look for Wolff's brand kasha in your better supermarkets or health food stores. Another wheat– and gluten–free alternative is *quinoa*, which contains more protein than most other grains; a staple of the ancient Incas, it remains popular in South America to this day. Quinoa (pronounced *keen-wah*) makes a tasty alternative to potatoes and can be used as a side dish or added to vegetables to constitute a main dish. Look for quinoa at *Trader Joe's* as well as at most health food stores. (For your interest, Whole Foods Market Gluten Free Bakehouse is a dedicated facility that supplies gluten–free baked goods to a growing number of Whole Foods Market Stores. Check their Web site at www.wholefoodsmarket.com.)

The Relation of Gluten Intolerance to Celiac Disease Via the Leaky Gut

Gluten is important to us because of the adverse effect it has on the mucosa of the intestinal wall. With persons who are gluten intolerant, it causes inflammation, damage, and breakdown of that protective barrier which soon has its debilitating effect on the autoimmune system.

Gluten is a protein with a fancy name (*amorphous ergastic protein*) and is found with starch in the endosperm of some cereals, particularly rye, wheat, and barley. There is no gluten in oats, but they often grow near each other in open fields and are often processed on the same equipment, thereby causing a possible contamination of the oats when and if they come in contact with one another. The safest bet if a patient has intolerance to gluten is to stay away from wheat, rye, barley, and oats, as well.

"Gluten is responsible for the elasticity of kneaded dough, which allows it to be leavened, as well as the 'chewiness' of baked products like bagels. It is the glutenins (specifically, high molecular weight glutenins) that are especially critical to gluten quality" according to the Wikipedia.

So, practically all those baked goods that most of us love–breads, cake, pasta, as well as soups–contain gluten in one degree or another. How can you tell if you have a gluten problem? Some people, especially children, may be allergic to it and never know it. There are, however, telltale signs of it that raise a big red flag.

Signs of Celiac Disease

Gluten intolerance is the major cause of celiac disease, which is characterized by a child's distended abdomen and a failure to grow. Stunted growth is usually observed early on and stems from lack of proper nutrients crossing the barrier because of the damaging effect of gluten on the intestinal villi.

Aside from those characteristics, it is often observed that the child may suffer a skin condition such as eczema or psoriasis or a combination of the two. Apathy, tiredness, and malaise often accompany gluten intolerance and must be addressed.

The name of the disease probably was derived from the fact that the celiac ganglion, otherwise known as the solar plexus, is located right at the spot that is often called the *pit* of the stomach, just below the xiphoid process at the bottom of the sternum (breast bone). However, *celiac* is the Greek word for *belly*. Signs are painful stomach bloating, cramps, diarrhea, and constipation. This will be addressed in the account of young Z.A. There can be fatigue, weight loss, and malnutrition. As mentioned earlier, a significant sign in the very young is that they fail to grow! Other more serious long–term consequences are osteoporosis, nerve damage, and even an increased risk of intestinal cancer.

According to the researchers at the University of Maryland, celiac disease is much more prevalent than previously believed. "It afflicts as many as 1.5 million Americans, or about 1 in 133 people, as opposed to the 1 in 10,000 estimated previously." (Tufts, April 2003, p. 8)

A simple blood test known as an EMA (anti-endomysial antibody) is done to screen for celiac disease. If it turns out to be positive, then an intestinal biopsy is justified. Personally, I should think that an Intestinal Permeability Test would also be called for, for further verification. (This test will be covered in Part II.)

According to Tufts University, "the only treatment for celiac disease is a gluten-free diet that requires avoiding wheat, rye, barley, and some-times, oats as well as the hundreds of foods and ingredients made with those grains or their by-products." (Tufts, April 2003, p. 8) That includes a lot of favorite foods like pasta, many breakfast cereals, canned soups, lunch meats—and, even ice cream!

There is another side to this story that I would think will be wel-comed by most with the problem. If you recall, the intestinal wall re-news itself in the healthy individual every three to six days. Therefore, if one disciplines oneself for about a week (ten days would be better), the individual should feel and know the difference. All things being equal, that alone could turn the tide.

To reiterate, I have often felt that not enough emphasis is placed on what a patient should *stay away* from in order to bring about an allevia-tion or even a cure of a health problem. We are educated to believe that we have to *take* something in order to get well. Has it ever occurred to researchers that what you *avoid* will bring about a healing?

It has been my experience to have encountered (apparently) differ-ent problems at the same time on the same patient. I have also wit-nessed the fact that when one problem clears up, in many cases, so do the others. (Such as the case of W.S.) The physiological explanation for such an occurrence would be a lifelong research project in itself. But as further evidence of such a claim, I offer the following account of a young boy, Z.A., who suffered signs of eczema, psoriasis, and celiac disease all rolled into one!

The following is his story, which should not only reach the heart of anyone who reads it but should also instill hope in those who suffer similar health problems.

The Classic Case of Z.A.

One case initially diagnosed as eczema came to me a few years ago. Seven–year–old Z.A. suffered the agonies of this disease, practically from the day he was born. His devoted parents did all they could to help their son. They had taken him to various doctors, hospitals, and numerous dermatologists and had faithfully followed through on every measure recommended to them. Z.A.'s condition continued to worsen. Three dermatologists said it was the worst case of eczema they had ever encountered. After years of prescribing one drug after another, the doctors gave up, admitting their frustration and failure. In other words, Z.A. and his parents were on their own.

Finally, his mother contacted me, because she had heard of my success with children suffering from eczema and psoriasis. Rarely have I ever been so moved by such a fine boy. With his skin peeling, oozing, and taut, he moved with caution, as though any sudden movement would rip his skin open. That, coupled with a bulging abdomen as taut as a drum, along with stunted growth, made for one miserable little boy.

We started our therapy using the same principles that I had used with all the other children I have treated over the years. What stood out in my evaluation of this young boy was that *he was always constipated!* He would move his bowels every five days, rather than the normal one to three times a day. This, in my opinion, was the first problem that had to be corrected.

I placed him on a high alkaline/low acidic diet, plenty of water and one to three tablespoons of pure olive oil per day. No sweets, no processed foods, no junk food. Only foods that were whole foods for the most part were permitted.

Slowly we began to see a change. His skin showed signs of improvement with the activation of his bowels. The use of natural cathartics (laxatives) was encouraged.

Young Z.A., trooper that he was, hardly ever missed a day in school. He forced himself to attend in spite of his physical discomfort. His classmates, in this case, encouraged him by their fondness for him and watched the changes that were taking place with personal interest.

About a year went by, and Z.A. steadily improved. But there was still something amiss—his abdomen, although improving, still remained distended. While all the other kids in his class grew taller, Z.A. seemed to be at a standstill.

It was then that celiac disease was suspected. The next step was to get him off all gluten products, especially wheat, oats, rye, and barley. His mother learned all she could about gluten free foods and recipes, and after using my cookbook as a guide, she taught herself how to cook specialty items.

It wasn't long before the change was dramatic. His abdomen became flat as a board, his skin regenerated to the extent that it was as smooth as silk without a blemish. He grew in height and caught up with his classmates. He was a miracle in the making. Z.A. showed such improvement that his teachers, principal, and classmates showered him with praise, amazement, and encouragement.

A few more months passed, and Z.A. was over his problems. His friends, parents, family, and teachers all treated him with adulation. Z.A. never complained through this two-year-long ordeal. Where many kids would insist on having the things they wanted, especially junk food, Z.A. never demanded anything. He knew what he had to do and he did it!

Three years had passed when out of the blue the producers of the *History Channel* called and requested an interview with me that was to be used in a special program featuring the life of Edgar Cayce. They asked that I provide at least one living example of a healing that took place by following the principles suggested in the Cayce readings. I chose to use Z.A.'s story as representative of the efficacy of the work.

His parents wholeheartedly agreed, not only to have Z.A. himself appear, but to have his mother appear on camera, as well. The filming and interview took place on a Saturday in August 2005, in my office, which ended up looking like a Hollywood sound stage by the time everything was set up. I was interviewed extensively, as were Z.A. and his mother. All aspects of the healing were covered, followed by close-ups showing the purity of Z.A.'s skin and a demonstration of my administering a spinal adjustment.

The producer and crew were ecstatic at the completion of the filming, which lasted all day. What a wonderful thing, I thought, that so many people, parents and children alike, would now see for themselves how they may be helped in cases of celiac disease combined with eczema and psoriasis. Such a filming had never been done before. We all waited with great anticipation for the day the program was to be aired. Sadly, our expectations were dashed when, two weeks before the program was scheduled to air, the home office of the History Channel wrote informing me that our segment of the program had been deleted because they had decided to focus on the *life* of Cayce rather than on his *works*. Needless to say my disappointment was great, as was that of Z.A., his parents, and his entire class who had all been eagerly anticipating the showing of the program. Z.A. would have won the hearts of anyone who saw the program and, more important, he would have given hope to so many sufferers of the diseases.

To this day the story of young Z.A. remains one of the most heart-warming cases I have had the privilege to attend. The following letters are among my most treasured reminders of what can be done in the healing of a fellow human being when one is on the right track.

Dear Dr. Pagano,
I'm writing this letter to thank you for helping my son Z. to heal from this skin disorder called eczema. Z. suffered so much for seven years. As you know Z. started with eczema at 1 month old. I took him to see so many dermatologists for the first 7 years of his life. One dermatologist gave up on him so he sent me to another dermatologist. Z. was put on so many different cortisone creams and ointments, also he was taking so much of antihistamine and steroids. I believe that due to all these medications, Z. did not grow as fast as the other kids grew. His skin was like an elephant skin, so dry and chapped. He couldn't sleep during the nights, he would wake up with blood on him and his sheets. His skin was so irritated that he would get infections with green mucus.

Today, Z. is completely clear of eczema and he is a 9½ year old boy who [hasn't taken] medication for 2½ years. Z. is so thankful to you Dr. Pagano and loves you for helping him.
Love, G.A.
February 17, 2003

Needless to say, such a letter is a precious treasure. The following is a letter from the patient himself:

> Dear Dr. Pagano,
> I'm writing this letter to thank you for helping me clear up my skin. I thank you from the bottom of my heart for helping me.
> When my skin was rough and bumpy everybody would make fun of me, and they thought that if they would touch me they would get it too. But today I have a lot of friends and everyone looks at me as a different person. Thanks to you.
> I thank my grandma, my mom and most of all Dr. Pagano. If I could I'd give the whole world to you. Thank you for all you've done for me and my family.
> Love,
> Z.A.

Because of its close correlation to this subject, the above was taken from the chapter on eczema from the sixth edition of my book *Healing Psoriasis: The Natural Alternative.*

This stands out as one of the most challenging cases I have ever encountered in my nearly fifty years in clinical practice. Without the strong support and determination of his devoted mother, G.A., such a result might never have taken place. A lesser woman might have given up hope or simply entrusted her son to the medical professionals, whose task, in this case, might have been impossible.

Instead, Mrs. A. took an active part in her son's recovery and helped reverse a devastating disease that he seemed to have been born with, taking him from a state of pain, weakness, and disfigurement to one of health, strength, and beauty.

If she never does another thing, she will have proven to all those sufferers of celiac disease that it can be, and has been, healed in a natural way. What it takes is the right procedure, trust, and above all, determination!

A year after our experience with the History Channel, I received a phone call from Z.A.'s mother, inviting me to a special function that they were having in honor of their son. Of course I accepted, and when asked if I would say a few words at the party, I willingly agreed.

I thought that I had already extracted all the possible joy that I could have from Z.A.'s healing, but I was wrong. While I stood in the wings and watched him dance up a storm, my eyes filled up, my throat contracted, and I could hardly breathe. He out–danced every child in the hall. As his friends threw him up in the air, he laughed until I thought that his sides would burst. Everyone was screaming and laughing joyfully at his gyrations.

What greater joy can a physician experience than seeing his patient, who, in the not too distant past, could hardly walk, move, or even breathe, and whose skin had been as taut as a drum—but now having pliable, smooth, and blemish–free skin and the unhealthy bulge of his abdomen gone!

Let me tell you, *there is no greater joy*—at least not for this physician. Young Z.A. proved by his dedication and sacrifice, not to mention the devoted help of his parents, that you do not have to live with this disease.

Some will call it a miracle, and so do I—but it was a hard work miracle!

PART II
Healing the Leaky Gut Syndrome

8

---•--•--•--•--•--

Nutritional and Therapeutic Considerations

Introduction

I t is the author's ardent hope that the reader by now has a clearer understanding of what is meant by the Leaky Gut Syndrome and how far reaching it can be. This section deals with methods, tools and principles on healing the leaky gut and restoring it to normal function with some examples as well as testimonials where appropriate.

Each topic covered in the following pages to the end of this book deals in some way with the suggestions that may be considered in the restoration process. Fortunately, practically every measure outlined lies within the power of the reader himself, is non-invasive and has few, if any, side effects. Nevertheless, anyone who wishes to follow these suggestions should not attempt it unless approved by his/her personal physician.

The following methods have one primary goal—*the restoration of the gut wall to normal function*. Basically there are five things that must be addressed in order for this to be accomplished:

1. Calm down the inflammatory process that has taken place to the intestinal villi as a first step in reestablishing the inner lumen of the intestinal wall.

2. Eliminate or greatly reduce the damage done to the gut wall by toxic elements and/or food allergens.

3. Reinoculate or "reseed" the small intestine as well as the colon with beneficial or "friendly" bacteria to the point where they exceed the number of toxic bacteria and/or other damaging microforms.

4. Build up liver function to make it more capable of carrying out the detoxification process.

5. Medically, Nystatin and Deflucan are two of the medications most often prescribed for yeast/fungi/mold overgrowth. This would have to be discussed with your medical doctor.

The following suggestions all aim to accentuate the healing process to one degree or another. There are others to be sure, so my readers should look upon the following considerations as perhaps the most popular but by no means as an exhaustive list.

Nutritional Considerations

1. Avoid the intake of foods and substances that have proven to be—or are even highly suspected of being—a food allergen or chemical insult to the gut wall.

2. L Glutamine and/or Glucosamine are food supplements that are proven aids in building up the gut wall. Others are: Omega 3 fish oils, Slippery Elm, Evening Primrose Oil, Cat's Claw, Milk Thistle (Silymarin) for liver regeneration and American Yellow Saffron Teas as a liver cleanser and intestinal antiseptic. (Note: Slippery Elm and American Yellow Saffron Tea should not be taken if a patient is pregnant or antici-pating pregnancy.)

3. Consume garlic and olive oil in cases of Candida Albicans (Can-dida), where yeast infection is proven to be present or even suspected.

4. Follow a high alkaline (80%) to low acid (20%) food intake. Learn what foods are alkaline reacting in the body and those that are acid forming and select accordingly. (These are listed in the Acid/Alkaline

Color Photographic Portfolio

The following photographic account represents a cross section of some classic types of psoriasis cases treated successfully by following the Cayce/Pagano approach to the diseases based on the Leaky Gut Syndrome (LGS).

The patients followed through with patience and persistence which brought about a successful result.

Permission to use these photographs has been granted by each patient or parent (in the case of children). Personal identification is omitted to protect the patients' right to privacy.

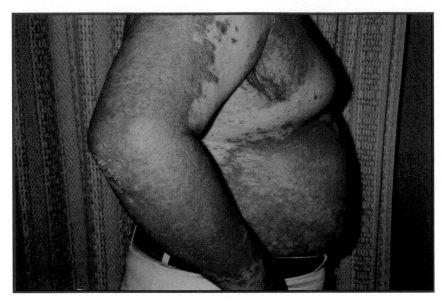

Start of regimen—right side

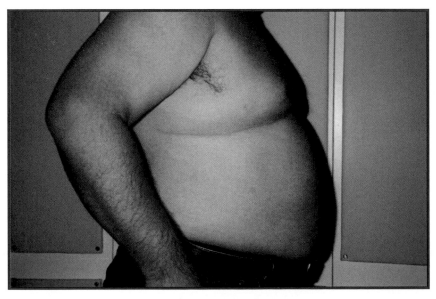

Nine months later

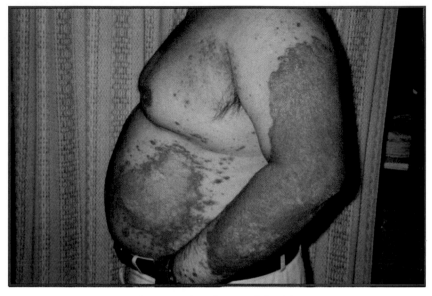

At start of regimen—left side

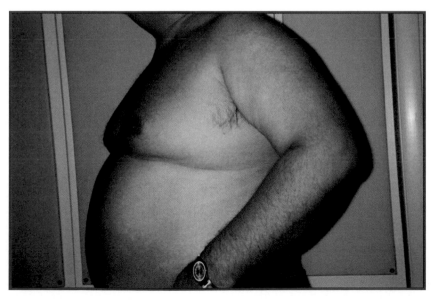

Nine months later

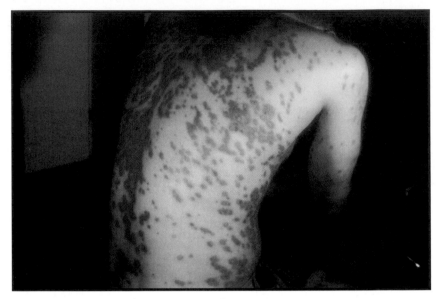

At start of regimen

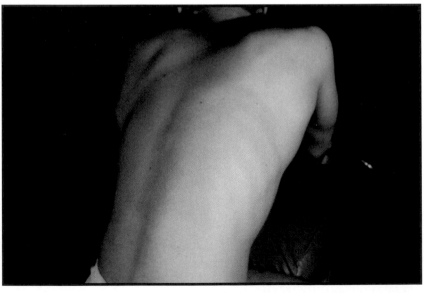

Seven months later

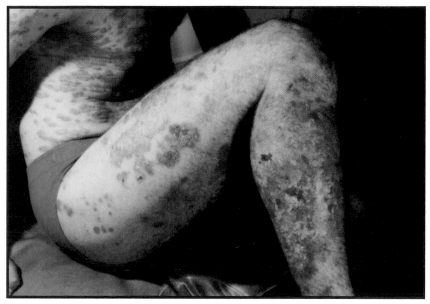

At start of regimen

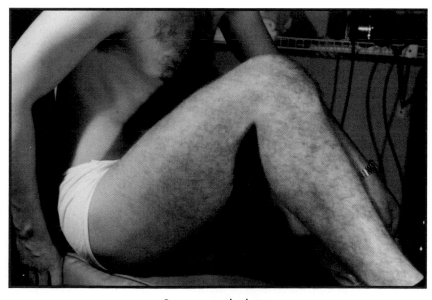

Seven months later

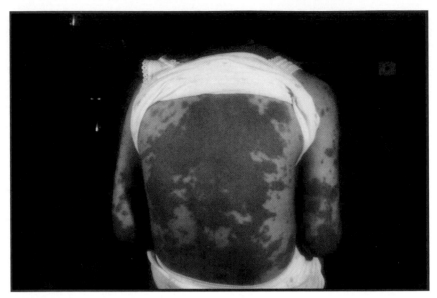

At start of regimen

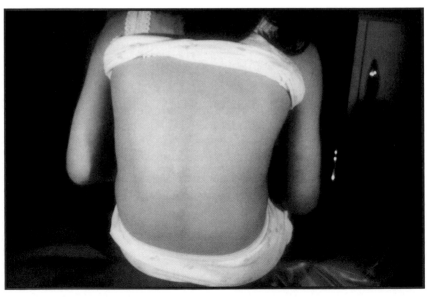

Less than three months later

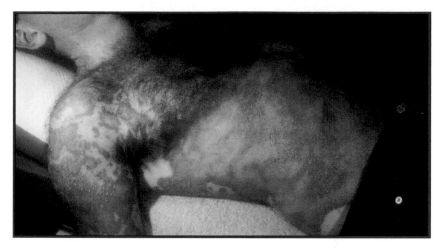

At start of regimen

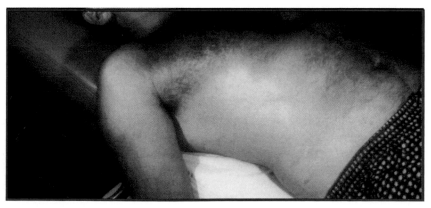

Eight months later

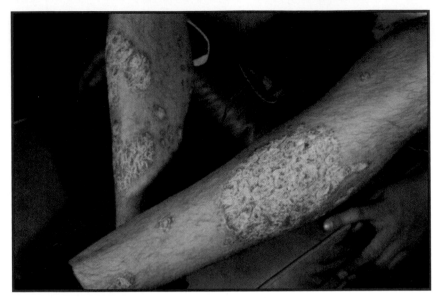

At start of regimen

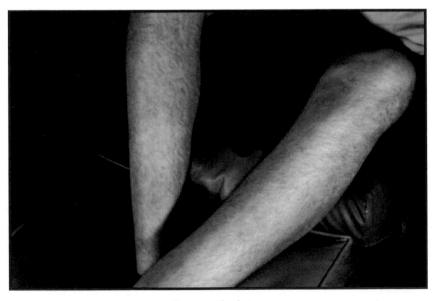

Six months later

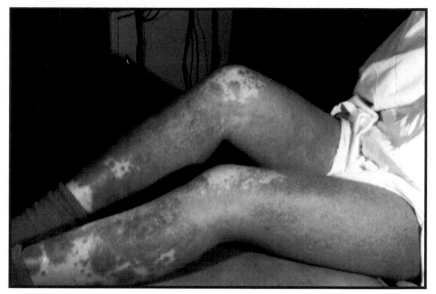

At start of regimen

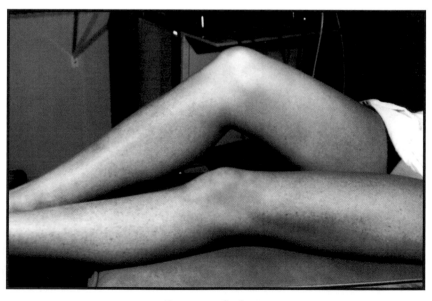

Four months later

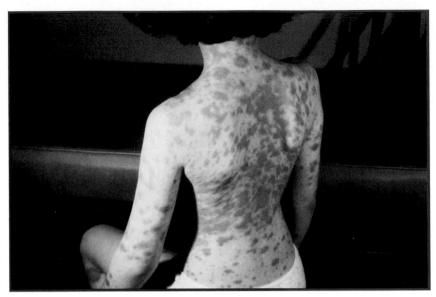

At start of regimen

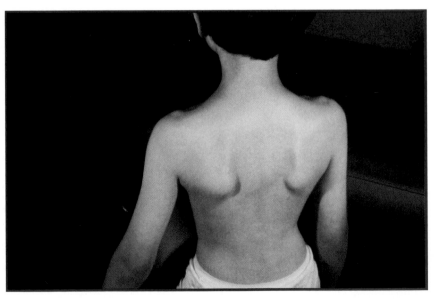

Two months later

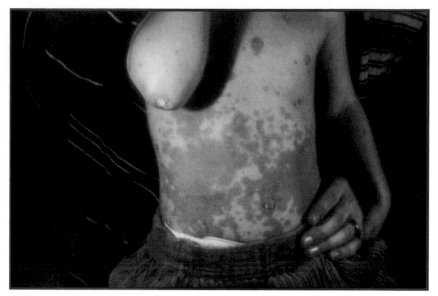

At start of regimen

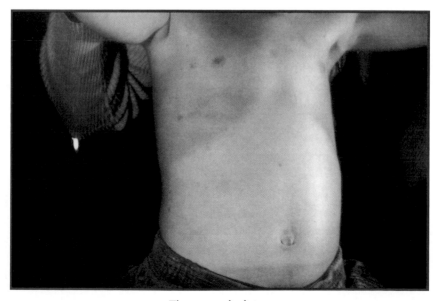

Three weeks later

The Herxheimer Reaction

The following series of three photographs is an example of how severe the purge period or *Herxheimer Reaction* can be in some people.

This reaction signifies that the immune system is in action throwing off the accumulated toxins that have built up within the patient, usually over a long period of time.

This sequence of photos shows the three stages of healing in this particular patient over a three-month period. Not all patients respond with this degree of severity.

However, when such a reaction does take place, it is imperative that the patient drink plenty of water and try to detoxify, including the use of enemas. This can speed the recovery time. This is the body's *die off* period when endotoxins are emitted through every pore of the skin during the cleansing process.

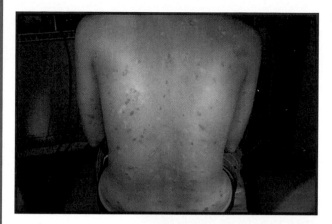

At start of regimen

One and ½ months later (the peak reaction)

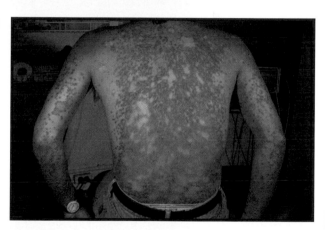

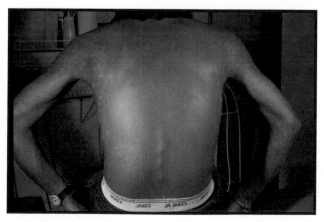

Three months after start of regimen

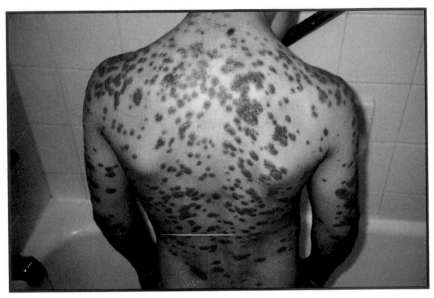

Young JJ— At start of regimen

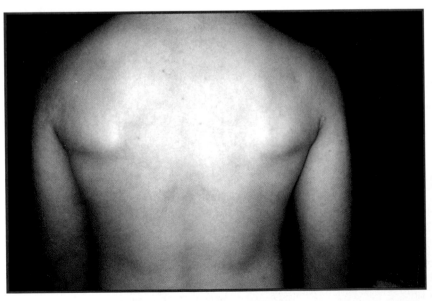

JJ—Seven and ½ months later

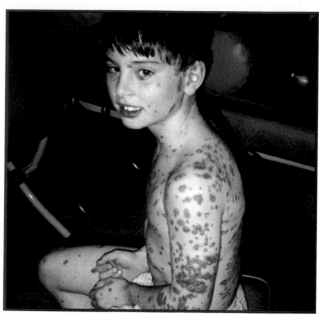

JJ—At start of regimen

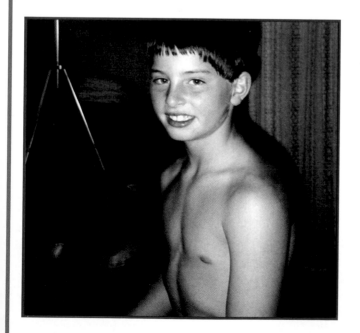

JJ—Seven and ½ months later

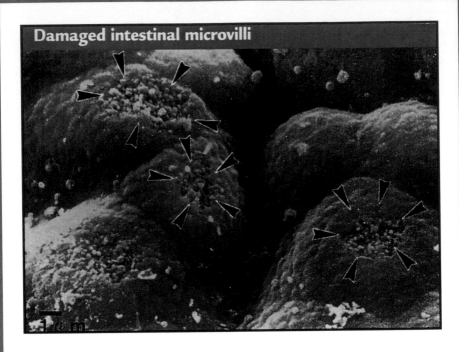

Damaged Intestinal Microvilli
[Reproduced through the courtesy of the Genova Diagnostic Lab]

Balance in a later chapter). The importance of this measure cannot be over-emphasized! Never consume any fried foods!

5. Limit the use of antibiotics, aspirin, and non-steroidal anti-inflammatory drugs (NSAIDS) as they damage the gut barrier and kill the "friendly" bacteria as well as the bad.

6. Reduce exposure to exogenous xylobiotics: i.e. pesticides, insecticides and irritant chemicals.

7. Eat more "organic" foods when available, especially when purchasing meats and dairy products. (See "A Word about Organic" in the pages that follow.)

8. Reestablish (reinoculate) the entire bowel with L Acidophilus such as plain yogurt with active cultures, to the point where the" friendly" bacteria outnumber the harmful ones, even if the count is in the millions or even billions.

9. Avoid sugars in all its forms especially if Candida (Yeast-fungi-mold overgrowth) is diagnosed or even suspected.

10. Increase the intake of fresh fish (ocean, wild-caught, is the best) They are rich in Omega 3 fish oils and vitamin A which restores the inner walls of the intestinal tract. Best are salmon, tuna, mackerel, herring, bluefish and sardines; the darker and oilier the fish, the better.

11. Increase foods with a high fiber content but be sure to drink plenty of water when doing so.

12. Drink 6-8 glasses of pure water per day. Fresh lemon or lime juice may be These are the basic dietary foods to consider, although there are others. So, with that as our starting point, let's move on to those measures that deserve serious consideration in helping to heal those inner intestinal walls where it all begins. You may find there is a bit of repetition. If so, it is by design, in order to drive the message home!

To Provide Additional Nutritional Support

1. Glutamine and L-Arginine—Both are single amino acids and have been shown to prevent and reverse gut wall damage from various attacks. *Glutamine is the principle fuel used by the upper intestinal tract and helps block bacterial invasion after the wall is damaged.*

2. Butyric acid—This is manufactured in the lower intestines as a

by-product of bacterial fermentation of fiber. It is the main energy source for lower intestinal and the colon epithelial cells. *It helps repair and regenerate damaged cells.*

3. Damage to the intestinal mucosa can be caused by oxygen–derived *free radicals* (known for the breakdown of body cells). Substances that help destroy the free radicals are: Vitamin E, beta–carotene, ascorbic acid (vitamin C), zinc, selenium, and superoxide desmutase. Most of these are *anti-oxidants.*

4. Anything that helps stimulate protective mucous secretions of the gut wall appears to be beneficial.

Therapeutic Considerations—Conventional Methods

Along with the dietary measures just suggested (with more to come), the following are listed as having a beneficial effect on LGS. Some of them you probably never heard of, some you may have. Even though you, as a reader, may be unfamiliar with them, I have chosen to list them anyway if only to expand your knowledge on the subject. Discussing these options with your personal physician would certainly be advisable.

The following are important because the condition of the gut wall is a determining factor in a person's systemic health pattern! *If the gut is not healthy, the person is not healthy.* The following substances have been shown to have a beneficial effect on preserving, repairing, and maintaining a healthy gut.

Lowering the Toxic Load

1. Bentonite clay—This is well-known for its ability as an intestinal absorbent of numerous toxins, endotoxins, and bacteria. Its value may be that it lowers the toxic load in the gut wall thus promoting repair.

2. Lactobacillus—This provides protection against increased permeability by building up the immune defense.

3. HCL (hydrochloric acid) and digestive enzymes. Pepsin, and pancreatin may diminish the antigenic and macromolecule load that approaches the gut wall.

To Counter Inflammation

1. Cromolyn sodium—This reduces increased permeability caused by ingesting food allergens. Quercitin, a natural *bioflavanoid* is molecularly similar to cromolyn sodium and also stabilizes mast cells. (Mast cells are cells found mainly in connective tissue.)

2. Gingko biloba—This has been shown to prevent the action of various substances that cause a deprivation of blood supply (ischemia) to the mucosal wall thus causing damage.

3. Prostaglandin E2 and E1—Prostaglandins are hormone-like substances derived from fatty acids and found in human body tissues and muscle activity.

The healing of LGS and regeneration of the gut wall using conventional methods or the suggestions by Edgar Cayce do not conflict, but rather complement one another. The scientific explanation of the pathology involved goes down to the cellular level, whereas, Edgar Cayce stops his general explanation with "There are those conditions, then, in the duodenum and through the jejunum where there are the effects as if there were tiny thinned walls, as if the walls of the duodenum had been smoothed . . . " (3373-1) From a practical point of view, actually that is all that is needed.

From a therapeutic approach, however, the procedures differ somewhat but with the same end result in mind—*to remove the antagonist and rebuild the walls of the intestine.* The following is a study of both points of view but with the same goal in mind, heal the gut, which in turn will heal the patient.

The Four Rs

From the *Functional Assessment Resource Manual* of the Genova Diagnostics Laboratory we learn the following, known scientifically as the 4 Rs. They stand for:

1. **R**emove
2. **R**eplace
3. **R**einoculate
4. **R**epair

Let's take a closer look at each one:

I urge my readers to read on even though some of the terms and suggestions are not familiar. You will find, however, that many are recognized by the average person. The more technical phrases may be explained to you by your physician or with a little research can be looked up online for technical assistance. The thing is not to get discouraged if you don't immediately understand some of the technical terms or words. Read on, and it will eventually all come together.

Remove the offenders.

What is there to remove? The answer is *the various culprits that brought about the problem in the first place.* It is pure common sense that as long as the irritant remains, the problem will remain. The first thing is to recognize what those culprits are and prevent their proliferation. In order to do this, consider the following:

• Remove mucosal irritants such as: allergenic foods, alcohol, gluten (if sensitive) NSAIDS (non–steroidal anti inflammatory drugs).

• Consider a Comprehensive Digestive Stoll Analysis (CDSA) or Comprehensive Parasitology, Bacterial Overgrowth of the Small Intestinal Breath Test.

• Reduce intake of sugar, refined carbohydrates, saturated fats, and red meat (meat can induce bacterial enzyme activity). Restore proper transit time. Increase dietary fiber and water.

Replace agents for digestive support.

• Consider pancreatic or plant enzymes, bile salts, betaine, HCL (hydrochloric acid), digestive herbs, or disaccharides (e.g. lactose) where needed.

• Consider CDSA, Lactose Intolerance Breath Test (or other disaccharide) to rule out disaccharide (enzyme) deficiency.

Reinoculate with friendly bacteria, if low.

• Consider CDSA, Microbiology, or Comprehensive Parasitology to rule out gut flora insufficiencies. (These tests are available through Genova Diagnostics.)

• Consider probiotic supplementation, including Lactobacilli and Bifidobacteria.

- Consider fructooligosaccharides (FOS) and inulin to enhance growth of friendly flora.

Author's note: Inulin (a form of insulin) is found abundantly in the Jerusalem Artichoke (Sunchoke), in onions, as well as in supplemental form.

Repair mucosal lining:

- Consider L-glutamine, EFA'S (essential fatty acids), zinc, pantothenic acid, vitamins C, E and A, beta carotene, N-acetyl glucosamine, gamma oryzanol, glycerin, and aloe vera.
- Consider antioxidants such as Vitamins C, E, and A, selenium, carotenoids, glutathione, N-acetyl cysteine, pycnogenol and flavonoids.
- Consider Saccharomyces boulardii, whey globulin concentrate or bovine colostrums to improve local immunity.
- Consider ginkgo biloba to enhance circulation to intestinal epithelium.
- Consider evaluation of overall nutritional status.

(For the benefit of the treating physician, tests are available through Genova Diagnostics, telephone 828-253-0621 or 800-522-4762. Genova Diagnostics makes it clear that the above information is presented for educational purposes only and is not intended in any way as an endorsement of treatment options.)

Elimination Diet

An *elimination diet* is one in which you identify, or suspect, the irritant(s) and stay away from them or eliminate them from your diet. I have seen this simple strategy work time and time again and thereby prevent exhausting and expensive remedies. Later, those same suspected culprits are re-introduced into the diet one by one, and the patient's reaction is observed and recorded. The patient keeps a journal for best results.

For instance, a seven year old female patient of mine suffering from severe psoriasis responded within a few weeks after she simply avoided a food item she absolutely loved, tomato ketchup! Her devoted parents took her to one of the leading psoriasis centers in New York City. In their evaluation of the child's condition, not a word was mentioned about diet. Her parents were advised, "Look, make your mind up; your daughter has psoriasis; you must bring her here twice a week for ultraviolet treatments indefinitely!" Needless to say the parents were devastated, not only because of the prognosis of their adorable child but the fact they lived at least a two-hour drive away from the hospital. It was on that same day they learned about my work and the natural approach I take with the disease.

An appointment was set at my office the very next day. It was there that I brought to their attention the vital role diet plays in the cause and alleviation of psoriasis. It was the first time they had even heard of the importance of food intake.

The problem did not reveal itself immediately but, after a month of no appreciable results, her mother one day inadvertently revealed to me that her daughter just loved tomato ketchup and poured it over practically everything she ate. She was the only one afflicted with psoriasis in a family of nine children. She was also the only one who gorged on ketchup! I shared with them the fact that ketchup is made up primarily of tomatoes, vinegar and sugar, three of the most powerful irritants of the gut wall. She immediately cut ketchup out of her diet. Within weeks the change was obvious. The next month her skin was free of all lesions—and she remains that way to this day, fifteen years later!

Therefore, don't be too surprised if it is but one item that's behind the LGS and by eliminating that item, the problem is often resolved. So there are certainly food items that cause LGS when used excessively over a long period of time.

Consider the following as possible suspects: The Nightshades—tomatoes, tobacco, eggplant, white potatoes (they are all white, except sweet potatoes and yams), peppers (except black pepper), and paprika. The nightshades are inflammatory foods, a good thing to avoid in LGS. (But more items to avoid later.)

9

───•──•──•──•──•──

The Yeast/Fungal Overgrowth: Candida Albicans

If a person has been diagnosed as having a "yeast infection" they think it stops there. But that is only a part of the story. That infection can spread through the blood stream and cause all sorts of problems which you would not think are even remotely connected to yeast overgrowth. For example, some of these are autism (as discussed earlier), ADD, ADHD, Tourette's, headache, depression, or even Alzheimer's—the list seems endless.

For a comprehensive report on the events that led to one couple's success over Candida after suffering for 19 years, I refer my readers to the true story of Mark and Alyson Cobb, chronicled on their Web site: www.candidafree.net. It is an inspiring story and all should read it for greater insight into the problem of yeast overgrowth. In their account, they convey the following poignant statements by Dr. William Shaw and Dr. Bruce Semon.

According to the Cobb Web site, Dr. William Shaw, scientist and founder of the Great Plains Laboratory, has a treatment protocol centered on prolonged doses of antifungal medications, including Nystatin, Lamasil, Sporanox, Nizoral, Diflucan, Caprilic Acid, grapefruit seed extract, and garlic extract. He found that the drugs worked as long as the patients were taking them. When the drugs were discontinued, the symptoms would recur. (Cobb and Cobb, n.d.)

Mark and Alyson Cobb further tell us about a "Dr. Bruce Semon, M.D., Ph.D., who has been treating yeast overgrowth with Nystatin and anti-fungals, had this to say: 'As long as the intestinal yeast is present and is making and releasing immunosuppressive factors, the body's immune system will have a difficult time clearing yeast from that area of the body. To clear yeast from that area, the yeast in the intestinal tract needs to be cleared first." (Cobb and Cobb, n.d.)

The natural way to clear the problem is a *change in diet*, and the use of probiotics—both of which are covered in later chapters of this book. The main object obviously is to attack the problem (whatever it may be) at the site of origin. Yeast/fungal overgrowth is one (if not the primary) factor that must be seriously addressed if results are to be expected.

Candida albicans is the organism that causes most yeast infections. In *The Yeast Connection Handbook*, William G. Crook states:

> "Based on clinical and research studies by many different observers, Candida overgrowth in your intestines may create what has been called a 'leaky gut'. Toxins and food allergens may then pass through this membrane and go to the other parts of your body, making you feel 'sick all over'." (Crook, 2000, p. 11)

Dr. Crook also makes it clear that "a diet rich in sugar and other simple carbohydrates prompts yeast overgrowth. Yeast overgrowth also can be caused by other factors, including:

- Hormonal changes associated with the normal menstrual cycle
- Birth control pills
- Pregnancy
- Steroids, taken by pill, injection or inhalation
- Genital irritations and abrasions
- Re-infection from your sexual partner
- Diabetes" (Crook, 2000, p, 8)

For anyone suffering from yeast overgrowth, or who suspects that one might be, this book and his classic *The Yeast Connection* are highly recommended.

As brought out in an earlier chapter, the body is always trying to help itself, and the repair of the inner gut wall is probably the most prolific anatomical structure of the body when it comes to regenerating. Once the gut wall has been diagnosed as being damaged, inflamed or compromised, there are, thankfully, things to do and items to take or avoid that will help bring about a replenished inner wall.

Yeast and Yeast-laden Products

The thing to do is starve the yeast. It thrives on many foods, but it craves sugar in all its forms more than any other food item. Some of the most powerful antimicrobial drugs and herbs are powerless against yeast.

You may recall how yeast, when locked in the convolutions of the small intestine, form fungus roots that penetrate the gut wall making it permeable to all sorts of waste products that find their way into the blood stream and consequently to every cell in the human body. Let's face it—we live in a sugar–saturated world. Sugar is in practically every commercial food item. So what do you do? You do the best you can. Read labels, avoid refined sugar especially, and keep natural sugars down to an absolute minimum.

Soft drinks rule the roost of liquid intake, especially among teenagers. Do you realize that one brand of soda contains as much as 12 teaspoons of sugar in one can! This is just one example of the overwhelming consumption of sugar in this country alone, and since sugar is the favorite food of yeast, it clearly has a direct connection with the development of LGS.

To repeat, sugar feeds yeast, and as long as the yeast is fed it stays nestled in the folds of the intestine. Remember that carbohydrates also convert to glucose (sugar) in the body.

Keep in mind, the best natural product to eliminate yeast is olive oil and garlic.

Sandra Cabot, M.D., author of *The Liver Cleansing Diet* also has a helpful Web site. On her site she discusses the liver and related diseases, one of which is Leaky Gut Syndrome. Dr. Cabot gives us the following information: according to the Analytical Reference Laboratories of North Melbourne, Australia, "If you can manage to eat 4 to 6 cloves of fresh garlic every day for 4 weeks, you will be amazed at the creatures that can be eradicated from your bowels. Garlic is able to kill bacteria, parasites, and yeasts." Their article goes on to say: "If you have a large overgrowth, even higher doses may be required. Raw garlic cloves can be grated, chopped very finely, or pressed in a garlic press, and then mixed well throughout your cooked food and salads. It tastes better with some cold pressed olive oil and apple cider vinegar. Raw onions and leeks also have valuable antibiotic effects in the bowel, and if you cannot tolerate garlic, you may find those things work well for you." (Cabot) It doesn't sound too bad, but I would think you should prepare yourself to lose a few friends along with the harmful microorganisms!

I include here two quick recipes to help include more healthful garlic in your life.

The Garlic Health Boat—a healthy hors d'oeuvre! Into a food processor is placed one drained can of chickpeas (organic if available), 2–3 cloves of garlic, quarter of an onion, 4–5 sprigs of parsley or cilantro, a quarter cup of olive oil, 2–3 tablespoons fresh lemon juice and some optional pitted black olives; the resulting paste is spread into celery sticks cut to 2–3 inch lengths, or eaten by the spoonful. A couple of the celery sticks or spoonfuls are eaten and the remainder is refrigerated to be consumed on several consecutive days. Not only is it truly tasty and enjoyable, it is thought to promote healing as well. Note: this recipe can be made using 8 ounces of store-bought plain or garlic flavored hummus (organic preferred!) in place of the chickpeas. As with any recipe, this one may be tweaked to produce the desired taste. For the average person, this recipe is an excellent cleanser for the intestines and can be done at every change of the seasons, i.e., four times a year. However, it is so tasty that many people enjoy it several times a month.

Nanette's Salad Dressing—Into an 8-oz. jar place 4 ounces of olive oil, 4 ounces of apple cider vinegar, 5–6 very finely chopped garlic cloves, ½ teaspoon oregano, salt and pepper to taste. Shake vigorously before each use.

Candidiasis (Yeast Infection)

To reiterate: yeast infections are due to a fungus. How can it be connected to LGS? Earlier it was explained that an overgrowth of yeast in the blood collects in the folds of the small intestine. Between the entrapment of the yeast and the gut wall that contains the billions of microvilli, a fungus forms and takes hold and begins to grow. The fungus grows roots (called rhizoids) that penetrate the gut wall creating the pinholes and breakthrough passages that compromises the lumen of the intestinal tract and renders it permeable to foreign or toxic elements. Unless that fungus is removed in the cleansing process, it will continue to spread its destructive effects throughout the body.

Remember, sugar is food for the yeast and fungus. It craves it and thrives on it—hence the need to discontinue taking it in. Once sugar is removed, the healing process can take place and renewal of the gut wall is the aftereffect. To help remove it, stay away from all sweets, including fruit juice for 2–3 weeks, drink plenty of water, and remember to eat the Garlic Health Boat.

We are told by Edgar Cayce to "keep the body alkaline" (1947-4) and that cold germs do not live in an alkaline system. They do breed in an acid or excess of acids of any character left in the system." Since sugar and sweets in general, are acid formers, prevailing alkalinity of the body would curtail yeast overgrowth as it does germs, viruses, and bacteria.

Quite profound in the Cayce discourses on this subject is reading 480-19:

> If an alkalinity is maintained in the system, especially with lettuce, carrots, and celery, these in the blood supply will maintain such a condition as to immunize a person.

Since LGS adversely affects the immune system and is classified as an autoimmune disease, I think the above suggestion should be given careful consideration as a formidable foe against yeast buildup.

10

·──·──·──·──·──·──·

The Immune System

In my search for a concise, easily understood description of the immune system and its close association with LGS, I was fortunate to come across an article in the Mayo Clinic Family Healthbook that clearly describes this vitally important system of our body.

> The job of the immune system is to protect the body from invaders that can harm it. An invader that prompts the body to produce antibodies is called an antigen (a term derived from the fact that these substances generate antibodies.) Antigens include harmful germs, viruses, and other foreign agents that can attack the body, and the immune system is vigilant in its search, recognition, and destruction of them. When the immune system recognizes a harmful invader and produces antibodies, these molecules circulate in the blood or reside in certain cells where they specifically counteract the invader. (Larson, 1990, p. 448)

Food represents the biggest challenge confronting the human immune system and since the surface area of the GI tract is greater than a tennis court, as Sidney Baker, M.D., postulates, it is the most active immune reacting surface of the body. How often have we heard the term "autoimmune disease"? We hear it often, but seldom is it explained. In light of the enormous surface area covered by the inner walls of the intestinal tract, concentration of the amelioration of any disease labeled "autoimmune" should be on the intestinal tract and the food that comes in contact with it. Since 60% of human antibodies are produced in the intestinal tract, intestinal permeability (LGS) compromises the body's immunity leaving the body susceptible to invading organisms of a viral or bacterial nature, or for that matter, any agent the body sees as foreign.

To summarize, an *antibody* is a protein molecule made by the immune system designed to intercept and neutralize a specific invading organism or other foreign substance known as an antigen. *Antigens* are mostly foods that trigger immune responses in the body. Generally speaking, they are polysaccharides (relatively complex carbohydrates) that are very large, often branched, molecules. They are sometimes called *glycons*. They are made up of starches, glycogen, cellulose, acidic polysaccharides, and bacterial capsule polysaccharides. To reflect a little, that describes what happens in LGS when the larger molecules of toxins breach the barrier of the intestinal wall and are interpreted and intercepted by the immune system as foreign invaders.

The Immunoglobulins (Ig's)—Antibodies

There are five immunoglobulins (Ig's) that roam our internal environment just looking for trouble. When a problem presents itself they go in to action, and what's so amazing, is that each has a certain, specific target that it goes after. The five immunoglobulins are: IgA, IgD, IgE, IgG, and IgM. Now that, I am sure, does not whet your appetite to learn more. But just think of it. Without them your body cells would be overwhelmed with the invaders who would literally destroy everything in their path. The Ig's are nature's "armed guard" that act on our behalf when called into action.

To illustrate, briefly:

IgA—this is the one most meaningful to us for when the gut lining is inflamed (LGS) the protective coating that is normally supplied by the IgA's is compromised and is not able to ward off protozoa, bacteria, viruses, and yeasts like candida.

SIgA—this stands for "secretory IgA." It is the predominant antibody or immune protein released by the body in external secretions such as saliva, tears and milk. It plays a major role in protecting the surfaces of the intestines by preventing the absorption of and/or disposing of microbial antigens such as germs and viruses and stops these pathogens from clinging to the cells and tissues of the intestinal mucosa.

IgG and IgG Complex are involved in 80% of all food allergy reactions.

IgE defends against parasites and is known as the *reginic antibody* for its major role in responding to offending foods and other environmental antigens.

Total IgE provides added insight into conditions such as eczema and asthma as well as inhalant and immediate allergies. It is believed that IgE antibodies trigger allergic reactions on the surface of the gastrointestinal tract when they crosslink with the GI mast cells. This causes a barrage of effects on the surrounding intestinal tissue and, by inducing intestinal permeability, *may also allow passage of food antigens into the bloodstream.* When this happens, other organs in the body become targets for the allergic reaction.

Admittedly, this is at best a briefing of the enormous job the Ig's have in maintaining the immune integrity of the human body. Several, as you can see, are directly linked to the care, maintenance and protection of the gut wall, and therefore are closely involved with the leaky gut syndrome.

(For a longer treatment of this important subject, see the article on "Antibody" in Wikipedia, the free online encyclopedia.)

What Are Allergies?

Briefly, allergies are the result of a response by the body's immune system to agents perceived as possibly dangerous to the body. It can be understood when you look at a gut wall which has broken down to the point that it can no longer identify the large macromolecules of toxic material. As mentioned earlier, the body's inherent defense mechanism views these antigens as foreign invaders and acts accordingly in the form of inflammatory reactions of one kind or another that can engulf the entire body.

Allergic foods add to the irritation of the intestinal walls and to a great extent they also prevent repair. Dairy and wheat have long been recognized as the most allergic reacting foods. In dairy it is lactose (milk sugar); in wheat, it is gluten (which is found also in oats, rye and barley.) Gluten is so highly allergenic, as previously explained, that it is the primary cause of celiac disease, causing malabsorption and malnutrition. The primary symptoms are gassiness, bloating and failure to grow normally. In celiac disease, for example, the millions upon millions of villi have collapsed and fail to absorb nutrients

Vitamin and Mineral Deficiencies

Earlier I mentioned there are two factors that enter this picture if a leaky gut is considered; that of *mineral deficiency* and, more likely, *vitamin deficiency* as well. One may take the recommended dietary allowances (RDA) of vitamins and minerals yet still suffer a deficiency of one or the other. The question is not only whether or not you are taking enough, but whether or not it is being absorbed! What good does it do to take them, either through your food intake or in supplements, if they never reach your body cells? This, I believe, is the origin of many neurological diseases the causes of which have never been determined. As mentioned earlier, some examples of such conditions are: multiple sclerosis (MS), muscular dystrophy (MD), amyotrophic lateral sclerosis (ALS), and even some conditions that seem far removed, such as autism, attention deficit disorder (ADD), and the elusive obsessive compulsive disorder (OCD).

Does this all seem far-fetched? I wish my readers to know that every one of the aforementioned conditions is found in scientific, medical literature as possibly having a leaky gut involved with the disorder. If this is true, how far can it go? I dare say, anywhere.

On Assimilation and Eliminations

Dr. McGarey relates: "In a case of diarrhea, Cayce saw the need for balance in the intestinal tract. He suggested that diarrhea resulted from the lack of proper food assimilation, or because of the introduction of toxic substances such as might be found in foods not normal to the individual." (McGarey, 1979, p. 82)

He goes on to say: "The Cayce material likewise recommends no solid foods at first, then gradually switching to a diet which eliminates starches for the most part. An alkaline–reacting diet builds resistance to such intestinal upsets. I'm sure that when Cayce made such suggestions he had in mind the Peyer's Patches, for those patches—in the context of the readings—are very important for healing, assimilating, and controlling the acid–base balance of the body." (McGarey, 1979, p. 82)

For a three–year–old who had diarrhea, Cayce gave the following suggestion: "Give small doses—a few drops of Glyco–Thymoline, in almost all the water taken. This as an antiseptic will keep down inflammation in the colon." (2289–6)

In case 2085 he suggested an immediate therapy of castor oil packs to the abdomen, along with a glass of water to which had been added a teaspoon of milk of bismuth and ten drops of lactated pepsin; the mixture to be stirred and taken slowly. At times osteopathic manipulations were suggested.

So the Peyer's Patches hold an honored place in the Cayce material. The rejuvenation of the entire body through these special glands by their re–awakening is certainly something we should all take into consideration especially since the method postulated is virtually safe: castor oil packs on the abdomen and Glyco–Thymoline (a mouthwash) as an antiseptic and alkalizer. Also consider American Yellow Saffron Tea as an antiseptic to the GI tract. (More on this will follow). *The only precaution that must be taken into account is if the patient is pregnant or anticipating pregnancy or if there is an allergy toward saffron tea and/or slippery elm. If either (or both) is the case, both teas should be avoided.*

Since these suggestions all have to do with the digestive system they will undoubtedly come in contact with all the structures and functions of the GI tract I cannot help but feel a leaky gut can easily fall into that category and the suggestions offered may have a beneficial effect upon the well-being of the individual.

To my way of thinking, one of the most profound discourses provided by Edgar Cayce is 311-4:

> There should be a warning to all bodies as to such conditions, for would the assimilations and the eliminations be kept nearer normal in the human family, the days might be extended to whatever period as was so desired: for the system is builded by the assimilations of that it takes within, and is able to bring resuscitation so long as the eliminations do not hinder.

In other words, if you eat right and absorb the food you eat, and have no constipation problem, you can live as long as you like! Not a bad legacy to leave us with, the rest is up to us.

11

——•——•——•——•——•——•——

Diagnostic and Therapeutic Protocols

Test for the Leaky Gut—*Measuring Permeability*

Earlier we touched upon the Intestinal Permeability Test which measures the ability of two nonmetabolized sugar molecules—mannitol and lactulose—to permeate the intestinal mucosa. Mannitol (small molecule) is readily absorbed and serves as a marker of transcellular uptake. Lactulose (large molecule) is only slightly absorbed and serves as a marker for mucosal integrity.

The test is a simple one. The patient mixes pre-measured amounts of lactulose and mannitol with pure water and drinks the mixture (called the *challenge substance*). The test measures the amount of lactulose and mannitol recovered in a six-hour urine sample, which is collected by the patient at home.

The test kit is supplied by Genova Diagnostics Laboratory through your health care provider. A complete list of instructions on how to carry out the test is contained in the kit along with all necessary supplies. Once your doctor explains it, you carry out the test as directed at home, then use the special mailing envelope provided to send two small

vials of your urine samples along with a nominal fee to Genova Diagnostics. The results, which indicate whether or not you have intestinal
permeability (LGS) will be mailed to your physician.

If there is a question as to the status of the gut wall, even after this
test, Dr. Leo Galland recommends having the test repeated for double
verification. If the test proves positive and you go on to a healing protocol (which will follow in a later chapter of this book), Dr. Galland
suggests you repeat the test in about two weeks to measure the possible
degree of healing. I believe, and this opinion is shared by many other
physicians, that this test is a godsend to patient and physician alike if
LGS is suspected.

(Ordering information for your physician: Genova Diagnostics, 63
Zillicoa Street, Ashville, NC 28801-1074, USA. Telephone: 828-253-0621
or 800-522-4762. Fax: 828-252-9303.)

A Good Question:

What if one has psoriasis (or one of the many diseases listed as possibly being related to a leaky gut) but tests fail to reveal a leaky gut?
How is one to think about that?

The fact is this might be the case. Let's remember that intestinal permeability (or leaky gut) is a reasonable *theory* or hypothesis. It is a concept fostered in the Edgar Cayce readings and theorized by medical
experts as well. If satisfactory results are obtained by following the
health measures described here, we can assume we are on the right
track, even if (in a few cases) LGS is not confirmed by clinical tests. In
other words, "If it works, it works!" No doubt internal pollution of the
body may have other origins. The thing to do is concentrate on purifi-
cation of the body, a measure that is almost intuitive and cannot be
refuted by any thinking person—scientist or layman!

Several possibilities come to mind. If the initial test for LGS was conducted several weeks or months after the patient started the regimen,
the leaky gut may have already healed over, yet the symptoms may
take longer to disappear. Or it may be that the test should be repeated
some weeks later to verify the status as Dr. Galland suggested earlier. It
may be liver congestion or colon impaction that caused toxic build-up
throughout the system without necessarily producing a leaky gut.

Whatever the case, if the problem shows signs of improvement, keep going in that direction. It has often been recognized and said that medicine (or healing) is not an exact science. A healing may take place without being explained by science as we know it. This has often been the case throughout history. If satisfactory results are obtained, let's just enjoy it and be grateful. Someday the scientists may get around to proving LGS one way or the other. In the meantime, let's just try to get well. The researchers will eventually catch up—maybe!

Castor Oil Packs—*A topical application for LGS*

To this point I have not mentioned any external (topical) applications that might be possible aids in the regeneration of the leaky gut. Is there such an application that may help this process? I believe there is—the Castor Oil Pack described by Edgar Cayce. Cayce suggested castor oil packs as a valuable health measure very, very often in his over 8,000 discourses on health matters. Castor oil held an honored place with Edgar Cayce, who called for its use in such conditions as arthritis, back pain, muscular and joint pain, contractions, spasms, gall bladder attacks and kidney stones.

I can attest to the efficacy of the last application, for kidney stones, from my own very personal, painful experience! When the kidney stone attack took place, I thought it was the worst pain anyone can endure. Being quite aware of the use of castor oil packs for kidney stones, I was eager to try this remedy for myself, but instead I was whisked off to the hospital by the police before I could even give the remedy a try. Once the diagnosis was confirmed I was placed on a strong pain-killer and hospitalized for seven days. The attacks came spasmodically. Each seemed more severe than the one before. At a period of relief (when the stone moved from one stricture to the other in the ureter) I talked my doctor into releasing me from the hospital with the understanding that I would return if the pains returned.

I had no sooner walked through the front door of my home when the stabbing pain returned in all its ugliness—but this time I had control. My mother had come to stay with me during my convalescence, so I asked her to make me two hot castor oil packs, one to be placed under my back, and the other on the front of my abdomen, both on my right side. Where the Demerol had taken 1–2 hours to numb the pain and then left me in a stupor, the hot castor oil packs gave me almost total relief in less than five minutes! This was repeated every day for a week and (with the additional help of a six–pack of beer my father slipped under my bed) I passed the stone. Ah, good old dad!! Of course, all evidence of having a kidney stone passed. Through the years I have recommended this remedy to at least three people who experienced the same results.

Most important to realize here is that castor oil, when applied in this manner, is absorbed by the pores and penetrates the skin, especially if left on for at least one hour, preferably two. It can make its way into the structures of the intestinal tract thereby nourishing the intestinal villi which will help dislodge toxic elements, such as yeast overgrowth, from the intestinal wall. That, combined with olive oil and chopped garlic taken internally, should bring about a decided benefit.

How does this possibly fit in with LGS? By virtue of the fact that the healing forces described by Edgar Cayce do in fact penetrate the skin, and where called for, can benefit the patient. This action of penetration of castor oil is extremely helpful when one understands the anatomical structure we spoke of as *Peyer's Patches*.

If you remember: "Peyer's Patches are best marked in the young, become indistinct in middle age, and sometimes disappear altogether in advanced life. Cayce readings suggested that these patches tend to become fewer in number as the body grows weaker, and that the regular use of castor oil packs over the abdomen tends to rejuvenate these glands and thus serve as a major factor in the rejuvenation of the entire body." (Reilly and Brod, 1975, p. 334)

Dr. McGarey, in referring to the importance of Peyer's Patches states, "Castor oil packs, one might postulate, could well have an influence on the length of one's life." If they are located in the lining of the small intestine as is illustrated in Gray's Anatomy, I believe it is safe to assume they are in close, if not direct, contact with the billions of microscopic villi that line the small intestine. With irritation of these walls, the Peyer's Patches are sure to be involved to one degree or another resulting in a deleterious effect to their function.

If hot castor oil packs over the abdomen help regenerate the Peyer's Patches, as Cayce suggests, it most assuredly must beneficially affect the intestinal villi as well, since they are housed within them. Admittedly this is theory, but knowing and experiencing the benefits of castor oil firsthand, I would say such a theory is based on a sound footing.

Castor Oil Packs on the Abdomen

Having studied and dealt with this application for so many years, I look upon this as a true healing procedure that may very well apply to LGS. This will not only benefit the Peyer's Patches, but the entire abdominal cavity which holds the small and large intestines as well.

In my practice with my patients, there are two ways that castor oil packs can be applied to the abdomen, the classic way, and the easy way. Let's start with the classic way.

The Classic Way—Materials Needed:

1. Castor oil
2. White cotton flannel cloth (such as an infant receiving blanket). The size depends on the size of the person. When folded it should be four layers thick. The average adult needs about a 16" x 20" piece of flannel, folded into four layers. (The size can be reduced for children.)
3. Plastic sheet of medium thickness. A clean plastic trash can liner about 30–gallon size is ideal.
4. Waterproof electric heating pad
5. Bath sheet or beach towel
6. Two safety pins
7. Plastic covers, such as those from the drycleaners

Procedure:

1. The flannel is placed in a small glass baking dish. Castor oil is poured over the cloth until it is saturated. (After use, the pack is kept covered in this container in the refrigerator for reheating as needed.) The pack is heated in the oven until it is warm, not hot, since it can burn easily. I do not recommend that my patients use the microwave since doing so might change the molecular makeup of the castor oil and

thereby reduce its effectiveness.

2. The plastic bag is placed on the bed to protect the sheets, and is covered with an old towel or cloth.

3. My patient lies on his back over the plastic and cloth and places the heated pack over his abdomen.

4. A plastic covering is applied over the soaked flannel cloth.

5. The waterproof heating pad is placed over the plastic, and the temperature is kept comfortable, not too hot.

6. A towel folded lengthwise is wrapped around the waist and abdomen and fastened with two safety pins. (A large bath or beach towel serves very well.)

(The above procedure is taken from the works of H.J. Reilly, with slight modification.) I advise my patients not to attempt it without prior approval of their personal physician.

The Easy Way

The above description was the classic way developed by H.J. Reilly and detailed in his thorough account *The Edgar Cayce Handbook for Health through Drugless Therapy.* (Reilly, 1975) The following is my version developed simply because the above seemed to be too troublesome to some of my patients, even though it is the best way to go. Therefore, to simplify:

Procedure

1. The materials are the same as above, but the flannel is replaced by a cotton washcloth, and a small Turkish towel is added.

2. Lying on the back, my patient liberally spreads the castor oil over the abdomen with the hand, rubbing it in very well.

3. The cotton washcloth is placed in a small plastic container and castor oil is poured over it until the fabric is saturated. (After the treatment, the washcloth is returned to this container, the lid is closed, and it is stored in the refrigerator for the next use. This cloth need not be washed out.)

4. The saturated washcloth is placed over the abdomen.

5. A hot, wet, wrung-out Turkish towel is placed over the washcloth.

6. A heating pad is placed over the hot towel (if the heating pad is

not waterproof, a piece of plastic wrap is placed over the hot moist towel before the heating pad is applied).

7. My patient lies on the back with the knees up and applies the heat for about one hour, if possible. (Everybody is different—a level of heat should be chosen that is comfortable for the patient.)

Whether using the classic way or the easy way, I believe it is beneficial to periodically place the hand under the entire pack and massage the abdomen. Plenty of absorbent paper towels should be kept handy to wipe the hands after massaging with the oils.

Generally speaking I have recommended that my patients use the packs consecutively for 3 or 4 nights then refrain for 3 nights. The actual castor oil pack never needs to be washed out; it is stored in a plastic bag or covered glass container and refrigerated until the next use. It can last from 6 months to a year. At each use, more castor oil is added for that treatment.

In my clinical experience, both procedures have proven to be beneficial for problems in the intestines, colon, liver and even pancreas. Again, do *not* undertake them without the approval of your personal physician.

Remember, the object here is not to attempt to live forever, but to live your life, however long it may be, in as good a state of health as is humanly possible to achieve. If we can pick up a few more healthy years in the bargain, I say "Let's go for it!" *It is not the number of years in your life that matters; it is the amount of life in your years that has real meaning!*

Castor Oil Packs on the Spine

In conditions of the spine, such as ankylosing spondylitis, psoriatic spondylitis, spondyloarthropathy and any other musculo-skeletal involvement of the spine, all of which may clearly be related to a leaky gut, the castor oil packs have in many cases proven to be a godsend.

You may ask why not in all cases? The answer, more often than not, lies in the discipline of the patient. Admittedly it can be a nuisance and bothersome at times, but the alternative of total freezing of the spine's mobility is far more troublesome, not to mention painful!

Years ago, a young postal worker in his 30s came to me with a spinal condition known as Marie Strumpel's disease. This is a spinal problem that begins in the lower spine/sacral area that becomes arthritic and slowly creeps up until it engulfs the entire spine rendering it totally fused. Unless stopped in its tracks, it eventually leads to total invalidism. The problem was there was no conventional remedy for it other than pain killers, which were increasingly being prescribed for him.

Since, for most arthritic conditions, the Cayce works often suggested the use of castor oil and/or peanut oil packs and massages along with an alkaline diet, I thought it might be of some help to apply them to his spine, in conjunction with spinal adjustments. The patient was given explicit and careful instructions on how to apply the packs, especially the castor oil packs on his lower spine, since x-rays of the area revealed the calcific changes completely surrounded the joints, cartilages and ligaments throughout the sacroiliac area on up to the third lumbar.

In about one month, during which I saw him once a week, we noted a decided change for the better. The treatments were working! Then, as enthusiastic as both of us had been to continue the procedure as long as was required, the patient inexplicably stopped coming. Weeks went by without a word from him. Bewildered and disappointed, I chalked it up to a failed attempt.

It was almost a year later that I unexpectedly got word of him from one of his colleagues. I asked about the status of my former patient, and his friend said, "He didn't come back, did he?" Fearing the worst, I said, no, but further explained that it seemed we were doing so well that I couldn't fathom why he would have stopped coming. The colleague responded, "I know why, Doc. He was getting well so fast that he was afraid he would stop receiving his disability checks!"

Shocking, isn't it? In my humble opinion, perhaps a person with such an attitude doesn't deserve to enjoy good health. Let him enjoy his disability checks instead of the flexible, functioning spine he might have enjoyed with proper treatment had he continued, since everything indicated that that's where he was heading. I wonder if those checks comforted him when his spine became rigid?

I still appreciate that case for it proved that the application of warm castor oil packs on spine and joint disease has the potential for remarkable benefits if the patient cooperates and disciplines himself to do what is required.

Procedure for Castor Oil Packs to the Spine
The patient lies prone (on his stomach) on a table about 30" high. A massage table works very well.

Warm castor oil is applied along the length of the spine, from cervical to sacrum. After massaging the oil deep into the paravertebral area, along each side of the bony protrusions (spinous processes) of the spine, a four-layer-thick white cotton flannel cloth, saturated with castor oil, is placed along the length of the spine. This is covered by a long piece of plastic wrap, which in turn is covered with a Turkish towel. Over this is placed a heating pad. (One of the best heating pads on the market today is the standard-size "Thermophore" with patient control. Smaller sizes are also available.)

The castor oil will penetrate and bring its healing effect to the areas it touches. Average time using the pack is between 30 and 60 minutes, with the heating pad on medium, never too hot for the comfort of the patient!

This procedure should NOT be undertaken without the approval of your personal physician or health care practitioner.

(Note: a complete *Castor Oil Pack Kit* is available through Baar Products, 800-269-2502.)

Castor Oil—Taken Internally

Castor oil continues to be the most common cathartic used by man. While this book thus far has emphasized its external use as a topical application, when used properly, it is without equal as a purging agent. The use of castor oil goes back thousands of years.

During a lecture tour in Bangalore, India, I learned a simple technique for taking castor oil internally that has proven to be quite effective. It is taking castor oil followed by a cup of tea. That's it! One swallows a teaspoon of castor oil, then immediately follows it by slowly sipping a cup of hot herbal tea, without the addition of milk or sugar. Any herbal tea will do, but it should be decaffeinated. If it hasn't worked in four hours, the procedure is repeated, and again in four hours until it works. (It could also be done in this manner with warm apple or prune juice, or another fruit juice if preferred.) The patient knows, better than anyone else, when it works! Once it has accomplished its mission, it is stopped, because castor oil can become habit-forming if taken too often. Over the years I have often suggested that my own patients who have a recurring problem with constipation conduct this practice once a month. Reliance upon one's own function of elimination is the desired goal.

Infantile Eczema—Hard to Believe, But True!

Were it not for the fact that I was the physician involved, I would consider the following account impossible or at least grossly exaggerated. Nevertheless, as a writer, especially one dealing in matters of health, I have the responsibility to tell the truth. The reader has the right to believe or disbelieve and I respect that. But I also have a duty to convey helpful information that I have acquired by study and experimentation or practical experience even if the message seems bizarre. Let's not forget the saying: "Yesterday's mysticism is today's science."

A call came late one Sunday evening from a patient of mine whom I had not seen for several years. She was not calling about herself, but about an infant, the daughter of her friend. The baby's parents were at their wit's end in trying to find some means to relieve their child's severe eczema.

If any persons wonder about the devastating effect severe infantile eczema has on a child and her parents, they should speak with the people involved, and they will find a heart-rending story which will make their own heart bleed. The parents hadn't slept in weeks because of the child's constant crying, scratching to the point of bleeding, persistent irritation, and rash covering her entire skin surface. They had taken her to a number of dermatologists, and had had her hospitalized once. Nothing seemed to work. The poor parents were left to fend for themselves.

It was at this point that my patient, whom I had treated for psoriasis many years earlier, learned of their dilemma and called me in the hope that I might be able to offer some hope. To be honest, when my patient called, I discouraged her from advising them to call me since I did not know them and the case seemed so severe. I was reluctant to take on another case of infantile eczema since it is too draining on everyone involved, including the attending physician!

I advised my caller that I had a full patient workload and would not be able to see them. Shortly thereafter, a second desperate call came from the parents themselves, and when I heard more of the difficulty this family was experiencing, I agreed to at least see the baby, but it couldn't be before the following Thursday since my appointment schedule was completely full.

Although they were disappointed, they agreed to wait the four days to bring the baby in for evaluation. Then they asked if there was anything they could do in the meantime to help their infant, especially with the intolerable itching which is the prime characteristic of eczema. "What to do?" I asked myself. My first impression was to advise them to seek another dermatologist or have the baby hospitalized—but they'd been there and done that!

While speaking with them I recalled an article by William A. McGarey, M.D., on infantile eczema titled "Healing Is Simple, Yet Magnificent" which had appeared in the magazine *Venture Inward*. Because I had been so impressed by the account I saved it through the years and was able to remember a few lines of this article.

Dr. McGarey related the story of an eight-month-old boy who had developed a rash when he was four weeks old. At first it was all over his body, then spread to both sides of his face. His mother told Dr. McGarey that he had been allergic "to everything I gave him." She related that she had not been surprised since there was a family history of the disease.

Dr. McGarey, author of *The Oil that Heals* and a strong advocate of the healing effects of castor oil, advised the baby's parents to use castor oil packs on his abdomen and to give him one drop of castor oil by mouth each night at bedtime. He viewed the problem as resulting from poor eliminations. Dr. McGarey reported:

> In two weeks, nearly all of the rash had disappeared. Food allergies which had been present since birth were gone. The

first week the rash worsened, then rapidly cleared. At the end of the period, just a faint memory of the rash remained on the left cheek. A two month check-up revealed that the child was healthy and clear of all signs of eczema. (McGarey, 1994)

Drawing on this information, I remembered two things, since I did not have the article before me at the time. The two factors I remembered were "eliminations" and "castor oil." Making no promises to the distraught parents, I passed on the information that eczema is a problem of poor eliminations and suggested they put a drop or two of castor oil in the baby's water bottle each night until I saw them on Thursday. Not surprisingly, they saw no logic in this, but having tried all medical options, they agreed to try it since there seemed to be no harm in the procedure.

May God be my judge, but on Wednesday night, the evening before their scheduled visit, the parents called to cancel the appointment because *the baby was clear of all lesions!* The parents were stunned—they could not believe that such results could be attained so quickly, and frankly, neither could I! But these are the facts. Was a leaky gut involved in this case? Possibly, especially when it is acknowledged that constipation is one of the recognized factors that have an adverse effect upon the intestinal villi.

"At the Hospital St. Vincent de Paul in Paris, permeability testing has been effectively used with allergic infants to determine which dietary modifications their mothers needed to make while breast–feeding and which of the 'hypoallergenic' infant formulas they needed to avoid in order to relieve their symptoms." (Galland, n.d.) This indicates that infants, as well as older children and adults, are not exempt from developing a leaky gut.

12

-•-⬤-•-⬤-•-⬤-•-⬤-•-⬤-•-

Dietary and Nutritional Considerations

The Acid/Alkaline Diet

'**ve** said it before and I'll say it again: "I have never helped a person with psoriasis, arthritis or eczema if they did not follow the diet!" All the other measures that helped bring about a successful result are important adjuncts to the healing of the disease. The spinal adjustments, herb teas, steam baths, enemas and colonics are all good and necessary, but without adherence to the Cayce/Pagano Regimen, results are simply not attained. Numerous dietary books have flooded the market in recent years, but only recently are the words *acid* and *alkaline* gaining recognition as an important part of health maintenance and disease prevention.

From the very beginning of his 45 years of giving readings on health, Edgar Cayce emphasized what he called the acid/alkaline balance in the daily diet. By this he meant we should eat 20% acid–forming foods to 80% alkaline–formers. Generally speaking, with very few exceptions the acid–formers are meats and grains and the alkaline–formers are fruits and vegetables.

There is another class of products, usually dairy, which some nutrition books classify as neutral, while others consider them alkaline. Diet-
minded researchers indicate they play a significant role in some people,
such as those suffering from eczema, arthritis and others who have demonstrated an allergy toward dairy products. It was, however, the acid/
base (alkaline) balance on which Cayce placed so much importance.
"Keep the body alkaline" rang through his works time and time again.

Simone Gabbay, author of the books *Nourishing the Body Temple* and
Visionary Medicine: Real Hope for Total Healing as well as many articles on
nutrition, writes:

> When the body becomes acidic, enzyme systems fail, lym-
> phatic function decreases, and energy slumps to a low. Cellu-
> lar metabolism is disrupted and toxins accumulate, making us
> less resistant to colds, infections and chronic illness.
> (Gabbay 1998)

Ms. Gabbay adds, in a personal communication to me:

> Probiotic bacteria promote a mildly acidic environment in the
> intestines, primarily through the production of lactic acid, thus
> keeping the growth of harmful, disease-causing bacteria in
> check. But while acids in the stomach and intestinal tract are
> essential for good digestion and the assimilation of nutrients,
> **they do not cause acidity in the rest of the body.** In fact, by
> helping to ensure the proper breakdown of proteins and min-
> erals, as well as the synthesis of vitamins in the intestines, they
> enhance the availability of alkaline-forming substances in the
> body. [Author's emphasis]

In the case of chronic yeast infection, for instance, sugars and sweets
feed the yeast. Sugar is acid-forming, therefore helps the yeast to thrive
and form fungi that penetrate the gut wall rendering it permeable to
toxic substances. A high alkaline diet will destroy the yeast and fungi
and aid in the repair of the gut wall.

Any biochemistry book will tell you that the blood should always be
slightly alkaline—that is, having a pH of 7.3 to 7.4. Yes, there are buffers
that help maintain that figure, but when the diet is so overwhelmed

with acid forming foods, you don't have to be an Einstein to know that the 80%/20% is fractured. The acids build up, the yeast thrives, the bacteria proliferate and the patient gets sicker and sicker with one disease or another.

To those readers who find this at least interesting and at most highly informative, I include here a list of acid and alkaline forming foods that I have used in my practice. Actually, this list can be helpful to anybody. Whole families have gone on this diet when only one member of the family had a problem that required a change in diet, and they have all been the beneficiaries.

70%-80% of the Daily Diet

70%–80% of the Daily Food Intake should be selected from the following, most of which are **alkaline** formers:

WATER: 6 to 8 glasses of pure water daily

LECITHIN: (granular) 1 tablespoon 3 times per day, 5 days per week.

FRUIT: (Fresh preferred, frozen is permitted, packed in water in glass jars on occasion.) Stewed fruits are highly recommended whenever possible.
Allowed: apples (cooked), apricots, most berries, cherries, dates, figs (unsulphured), grapes, grapefruit, lemons, limes, mango, nectarines, oranges, papaya, peaches, pears, pineapple, prunes (small), raisins, kiwi
Permitted in lesser quantities are: avocado, cranberries, currants, large prunes and plums.
Note: Raw apples, bananas, and melons are permitted, provided they are eaten alone and sparingly. In cases of candida, celiac disease, and other yeast–related problems, fruit and fruit juices are to be avoided for the time being.

VEGETABLES: Vegetables should be consumed more than fruits. At 2 to 3 fruits per day, 5 to 6 vegetables should be eaten. (Daily intake should be three that grow above the ground to one that grows below the ground. Fresh preferred, frozen permitted, packed in glass jars on occasion.)

Allowed: asparagus, beets, broccoli, Brussels sprouts, cabbage, carrots*, celery*, cucumbers, garlic*, lettuce* (romaine in particular), onions*, olives, parsnips, scallions, soy beans, spinach*, sprouts*, string beans, squash, sweet potatoes, watercress*. *Note:* Those marked with (*) are particularly important.

Note: Carrots and beets should be avoided in any yeast problem.

Permitted in lesser quantities are: corn (white corn preferred), dried beans, peas, lentils, rhubarb. Almonds are the only nuts that are alkaline. Eating five to ten raw almonds a day is suggested. Filberts are permitted occasionally.

JUICES: Vegetable and fruit juice daily (freshly made preferred) is highly recommended. A juicer and blender are the most valuable kitchen appliances a person should invest in.

20%-30% of the Daily Diet

20%–30% of the Daily Food Intake should be selected from the following, most of which are **acid** formers:

GRAINS: All grains should be *natural whole grain products* such as: breads, bagels, muffins, cereals with very little, if any, preservatives or artificial sweeteners. Rice (brown and/or wild preferred). *No white flour products.*

MEATS: **Fish** (Not shellfish) salt or fresh water (fresh or frozen). If canned, water or oil packed is permitted. Fish is beneficial, but, dark-fleshed, oily fish carries the most Omega–3 fatty acids, which are highly desirable. Wild is best!
Fowl (Poultry): chicken, turkey, Cornish hen, non–fatty wild fowl. (All skinless, white meat preferred)
Lamb: Trimmed of all fat before cooking, well done, once or twice a week.
Note: The above listed meats are never to be fried. No more than 4 to 6 oz. is permitted at a serving, once a day, unless the person has a heavy

work load or is very large in stature.

DAIRY: Only low fat/low sodium products are permitted: Skim or low fat milk, cheese, buttermilk, yogurt, etc. (No ice cream, cream toppings or whole milk products). Do not have citrus fruits or citrus juices with dairy products or cereals at the same meal.
Note: In cases of eczema: goat's milk and soy milk are suggested.

Butter (unsalted) is permitted but only occasionally and in very sparing amounts. (Even though it is a saturated fat, a little butter is better than margarine and other hydrogenated products).

Organic or free-range eggs are permitted, 2–4 per week, prepared any way but fried.

OILS: *Permitted:* olive oil, canola, safflower, cottonseed, soy bean, sunflower, sesame and occasionally peanut. One teaspoon of olive oil three times per day is suggested for most patients unless there is a gallbladder problem.

It is important to adhere to the 70–80% / 20–30% food selection in order to maintain a proper acid/alkaline balance. However, if this is found to be too difficult, a person should at least try to consume as many items in as large a variety as possible from the 70%–80% list.

AVOID
1. **Almost all saturated fats, such as:** red meats (except lamb): beef, pork, veal, sweetbreads, etc; processed meats: sausage, salami, bologna, frankfurters, hamburgers; hydrogenated products: margarine.

2. **The nightshades**: tomatoes (and tomato sauces and products), tobacco (smoking), eggplant, peppers (all types), white potatoes, paprika. Avoid hot spices of all kinds.

3. **Shellfish**: lobster, shrimp, clams, crabs, etc., and sauces made with shellfish.

4. **Junk Food**: soda (diet and regular), sweets, candy, pastries, chocolate (and all products made with chocolate), potato chips, French fries, etc.

5. **Yeast** or yeast laden foods: if there is an underlying yeast infection (Candidiasis).

6. **Miscellaneous**: All fried foods, pizza, alcohol (including beer), sugary cereals, wine or grain vinegar, pickled and smoked foods, hot spices, gravies, coconut, coconut oil, palm oil, mushrooms, and too many starches.

Note: In every case of psoriatic arthritis, avoid citrus fruit, strawberries and adding salt to foods. Salt in particular should be avoided at all costs. The salt (sodium) found naturally in the daily diet is quite adequate.

Avoiding the Nightshades

When you think of arthritis of any kind, think also of the nightshades. Arthritis, especially rheumatoid, is listed in many medical sources as being an offshoot of LGS. To repeat, the nightshades are: tomatoes, tobacco, eggplant, white potatoes, peppers, and paprika. These six members of the Solanaceae family of plants are believed to be the triggering mechanism for many aches and pains as well as irritants to skin problems. They literally carry a poison and in ancient times were sometimes given to the enemy in the hope that they would be consumed, render the enemy sick, and possibly even cause their demise at night—thus the term "nightshade."

Patients often ask what it is about the nightshades that make them undesirable especially to the psoriatic arthritic patient. To answer, I turn to the monumental work of Dr. Norman F. Childers, retired former professor at the University of Florida (Gainesville), founder of The Arthritis Nightshades Research Foundation, and author of *Arthritis: Childers' Diet that Stops It!* Dr. Childers is the leading authority on the nightshades and the devastating effect they can have on some individuals, especially those prone to psoriasis, psoriatic arthritis, and eczema.

By observation and by questioning my patients suffering from arthritis and/or psoriatic arthritis, I have learned that often the night-shades constituted a significant part of their diet. In fact many listed them among their favorites, especially tomatoes and peppers. When I placed them on a no–nightshades diet, as researched and taught by Dr. Childers, we saw results that could not be denied.

The nightshades are inflammatory foods that undoubtedly have an irritating affect on the intestinal villi of the small intestine, especially if consumed heavily on a regular basis. But why is it so hard for a patient to believe this? Probably for two reasons: first, they don't *want* to believe it; and second, it has never been taught to them. I favor the second explanation over the first.

Have you ever wondered why you have stiffness and pain in your joints when you get up in the morning, especially after you have had a meal composed largely of nightshades the night before?

Dr. Childers explains it as follows:

> There is an enzyme in muscles that gives us agility of movement, known as *cholinesterase*. Any chemical or factor that inhibits this enzyme will cause stiffness and soreness when it builds in our system to a critical level. Older people seem unable to counter this situation as well as younger people, but the latter are not entirely exempt. Cholinesterase inhibitors in the nightshades are: *solanine* in potato and eggplant, *tomatine* in tomato, *capsicum* in peppers and *nicotine* in tobacco.
> (Childers, 1984)

If the nightshades can do that to the human body, is there any doubt they can be a major player in compromising the intestinal wall? (For more information about Dr. Childers and his work or to order his book, visit his Web site at www.noarthritis.com.)

To this day the medical establishment refuses to believe that diet has anything to do with psoriasis in spite of all the evidence to the contrary. They are, however, slowly coming around to see the diet connection with arthritis, probably because of public demand and the ever–growing popularity of alternative or complementary medicine. Leaders in the field of medicine are speaking out as never before on the value of natural healing. Dr. James F. and Mrs. Balch's comprehensive book *Pre-*

scription for Nutritional Healing; the works of Andrew Weil, M.D. and Deepak Chopra, M.D., as well as the Cayce classic *The Edgar Cayce Handbook for Health through Drugless Therapy* by Reilly and Brod are examples of such ground-breakers. The movement is marching on and there is no stopping it—in spite of all efforts to quell its advance.

The Taking of the Teas

The importance of taking specific herbal teas in this approach to healing a leaky gut cannot be overemphasized. The purpose of taking the teas is twofold: 1) the healing of the inner walls of the intestines, and 2) the flushing out or cleansing of the alimentary canal.

1) Slippery Elm Bark Powder is used for healing the walls of the intestines. It is prepared by putting about a ¼ to ½ teaspoon of the powder in a cup of warm water and allowing it to steep for about 15 minutes. Stir occasionally and sip down. This is to be done in the morning, 30 minutes before breakfast. If for any reason this timing is not possible, it may be taken just before retiring the night before. It is taken five days out of the week for about 10 days; then every other day until the condition clears. If it seems difficult to take, add ice to the mixture—the colder the better. The slippery elm is also available in the form of capsules or Thayer's Lozenges, and they now come in different flavors which children prefer. In the event that the slippery elm bark powder is difficult to take, the capsules or lozenges are an acceptable alternative.

Women who are pregnant or are anticipating pregnancy should not take this tea. Omega 3 fish oils or flaxseed oil make an excellent substitute in the healing of the intestinal walls. (See below).

2) The American Yellow Saffron Tea (not Spanish) is for the purpose of flushing out the liver and kidneys. About ¼ to ½ teaspoon of the tea is placed in a cup and hot water is added. Let it steep for about 10 to 15 minutes, then strain and drink. It is best taken between meals or on a relatively empty stomach. Two or three cups can be had if desired—but there is one hard and fast rule to follow: *Do not drink the Slippery Elm Tea and the American Yellow Saffron Tea too close to each other. They should be taken at opposite ends of the day from each other.* Again, in cases of pregnancy or anticipated pregnancy, this tea should not be taken.

Saffron Water: A very cleansing and healthful measure is to prepare a gallon of saffron water and keep it in the refrigerator at all times. Bring a gallon of pure mountain spring or distilled water to a boil. Turn off the heat and add one full teaspoon of the saffron to the water and allow it to steep for about 20—30 minutes. Strain it and return it to the container the water originally came in, then refrigerate it. At least one full glass of this water is taken each day as part of your 6—8 glasses of water. It is a most effective way to flush out the system.

The taking of **Omega 3 Fish Oils** and/or **Flaxseed Oil** five days out of the week has been added to my regular regimen in the past few years, since they have been recognized as being very effective in the regeneration and reconstruction of the intestinal walls, thus helping to repair the "leaky gut." These, as well as L–Glutamine, may help considerably in this function, particularly when the breakdown of these walls can be traced to excessive use of antibiotics or drugs used in psoriasis such as Methotrexate (MTX).

These items, the teas and oils, should be kept refrigerated at all times while in their packages. They may be obtained from any well–supplied natural health food store. The American Yellow Saffron Tea is sometimes difficult to find. For both Slippery Elm Bark Powder and American Yellow Saffron Tea my patients deal directly with their health food store or a product supplier, such as Baar Products 1–800–269–2502.

Note: These teas may be taken provided they do not interfere with the absorption of any medication such as heart medication or diabetes. Always seek the advice of your licensed health practitioner for any contraindication before taking these teas.

The "YES" and "NO" Food Selections

Since the primary focus of attention regarding LGS is food intake, notwithstanding the part lifestyle and emotions play, I thought it might be helpful to list foods to avoid and foods to indulge in. These lists have been compiled from various authors and articles whose interest focused on LGS.

Here, at a glance, are the foods that should be avoided and those that may be enjoyed. I have chosen to use the simple words "Yes" and "No" to indicate what foods are acceptable and helpful, and which are not.

This list is by no means exhaustive since it is not possible to list every known food item that is available. It does, however, name the primary foods which are beneficial or deleterious.

The "NO" Foods—Avoid them!
Sugar
Alcohol (all kinds)
Red meat
The nightshades (tomatoes, tobacco, eggplant, white potatoes, peppers, paprika)
Ketchup
White bread (and white flour products)
Donuts, cookies, pastries
Soft drinks (diet or regular soda)
Candy, especially chocolate
Ice Cream
Pizza
Mushrooms
Vinegar (white or red)
Carrot juice
Beet juice
Coffee with cream and sugar
Wheat, oats, rye, or barley (if gluten intolerant or if celiac disease is suspected)
Most dairy products
Fermented foods
Corn
Peanuts
French fries and potato chips
Fried foods of any kind
Fried chicken or fish
Hot spices
Shellfish

Other factors to avoid:
Poor diet with high fat or sugar content

Smoking
Constipation (1–3 bowel movements a day is normal for everyone)
Any food item you know you are allergic to
Inflammatory foods such as the nightshades, sugar, hot spices, and gluten

The "YES" Foods—Enjoy them!
Water, pure, 6–8 eight-ounce glasses or half a gallon per day*
Olive Oil
Raw garlic
Green leafy vegetables and their juices
Raw vegetables and fruits (vegetables should outnumber fruits 4 to 1)
Fish, wild, cold, salt water varieties; and especially those high in omega
    3 such as salmon, tuna, mackerel, sardines, herring and bluefish
Chicken, organic, not fried
Turkey and wild fowl
Yogurt, plain with *active cultures*
Kefir, plain with *active cultures*
Buttermilk, with *active cultures*
Soy yogurt, plain with *active cultures*
Fresh lemon and lime
Onions, leeks, scallions and shallots
Raw ginger
Mild spices
Whole grain breads (in limited quantity)
Apple cider vinegar
Coffee, black, decaf (no more than 2 cups/day)
Almonds
Fiber foods (and/or supplements with plenty of water)
Aloe vera juice
    *unless there is a problem with urinary incontinence

Other Favorable Factors to Include:
Psyllium husks (or powder)
Probiotics—lactobacillus acidophilus, bifidobacterium
80%–20% alkaline–acid diet. Alkaline forming foods must override the
acid formers.

Foods steamed, broiled, baked, grilled, poached, etc., but not fried!

Note: Patients should try to concentrate and focus on foods they can have rather than those they should avoid. Obviously a person who is allergic to any of the "yes" foods should avoid them! This will save them from a sense of deprivation. Maintaining a positive outlook is crucial.

A Quick Review
The Deadly Seven
As was mentioned earlier, oftentimes a patient clears up a problem by simply staying away from certain food items. Through the years in my practice dealing with LGS I came to list what I call the Deadly Seven. It would be well if my readers would take the following seriously on foods and products to avoid:

1. Red meat and all processed meat (lamb is the only exception)
2. The nightshades: tomatoes (and tomato products), tobacco, eggplant, white potatoes, peppers and paprika
3. Too many sweets: products made with refined sugar, candy, chocolate, pastry, pizza, white flour products
4. Alcohol
5. Smoking (tobacco is a nightshade)
6. Fried foods (all fried foods) especially deep fried; French fries are one of the worst
7. Junk foods (refined sugar products, regular and diet soda, fast foods, potato chips, white bread, etc.)

The Glorious Seven
Here are the winners, the food items that can spell success in cases of LGS.

1. Water—fresh—six 8-ounce glasses a day. (You may add fresh lemon or lime juice.)
2. Vegetables—green leafy in particular, as well as tubers. The ratio of these vegetables should be three that grow *above* the ground to one that grows *below*. Keep the acid/alkaline balance. Vegetables and fruit should be 80% of the daily diet.
3. Fruit—fresh—they are the body cleansers. They are to be avoided, however, in cases of Candida and yeast-fungi overgrowth.
4. Fish, fowl and lamb—as animal protein. (Vegetarians should consider that brown rice and beans combine to make a complete protein.) These should constitute 20% of the daily diet.
5. Probiotics (yogurt, kefir) with active cultures.
6. Olive oil, garlic, and lemon juice, especially in cases of Candida.
7. Whole grain breads only—but not too much, as they are acid forming.

Read labels: pick products with the lowest count of carbohydrates (which convert to sugar) and sugar content. This may seem hard for some people to do. It's a matter of where you place your priorities. Do you want to get well or not? The answer to that (which only the patient can provide) determines your future in matters of health.

A Word About "Organic"

From the US Department of Agriculture (USDA) we learn specific guidelines to help consumers understand organic labeling.

Organic meats, poultry, eggs and dairy products come from animals that are given no antibiotics or growth hormones. This is good to know for everyone, but in particular for pregnant women, children, and people recovering from cancer.

Organic produce and grains are grown without the use of conventional pesticides, synthetic fertilizers, bio–engineering, or radiation.

From the USDA:

• Products labeled "100% Organic must contain *only* organic ingredients and may display the USDA seal. These are the *only* products which may display the USDA seal.

• Products labeled "Organic" must contain at least 95% organic ingredients. The other 5% (excluding water and salt) must be nonagricultural substances on an approved list, or non–organic products that are not available commercially in organic form. These products may *not* display the USDA seal.

• Products labeled "Made with Organic Ingredients" are processed food products (cereals, pastas, breads, canned goods, etc.) that must contain at least 70% organic ingredients. These products may *not* use the USDA seal.

• Processed products that contain less than 70% organic ingredients can list those ingredients as organic but cannot be labeled "organic."

The USDA advises that "organic" on a label does not guarantee a product that is "healthy." Be aware of calorie content and fat content.

To learn more, visit the Web site of the National Organic Standards Board at www.ams.usda.gov/nosb/ or the site of the National Organic Program at www.ams.usda.gov/nop/indexNet.htm. (Tufts, 2006)

It goes without saying that this is important information because "organic" foods have a more beneficial effect upon the body than do the non–organics which can be loaded with pesticides, fertilizers, and any number of harmful substances that find their way to the intestinal wall the moment they are consumed. As mentioned earlier, any substance that can cause damage to the gut wall can bring about the leaky gut syndrome.

Another Side of "Organic"

When something "new" comes on the market and proves itself to be desired by the public, everybody wants to get on the proverbial bandwagon and get a share of the action and the profits. The "organic" situation is a case in point. Lately, marketers are beginning to indiscriminately slap the "organic" on just about anything simply because they know that's what the public wants to buy.

The October 16, 2006, issue of *Business Week* carried the following cover article: "The Organic Myth" by Diane Brady. The subtitle, which appeared right on the front cover of the magazine, reads: "As it goes mass market, the organic food business is failing to stay true to its ideals," which is basically the message of the report. One revealing statistic she disclosed is the following: "The corporate giants have turned a *fringe food category* into a $14 billion business." (Brady, 2006, p. 54)

I recently heard a TV news item that actually referred to "organic" potato chips; I wouldn't be surprised if soon they will be promoting "organic" junk food as well! So, look for the organic label, but as always, *caveat emptor*—let the buyer beware! One can only hope that those who abuse the labeling guidelines and take advantage of the public to line their own pockets will one day be brought to task!

Probiotics

Lactobacillus acidophilus live primarily in the small intestines, *bifidobacterium* live primarily in the large intestine. They are called *probiotics* and are very healthful in reestablishing the "friendly" bacteria as the dominant factor in both the small and large intestine.

Sources of lactobacillus acidophilus are yogurt and kefir, which contain live, active cultures.

Also an aid to promote growth and proliferation of friendly bacteria is the probiotic *fructooligosaccharides*, known as FOS. FOS are not metabolized. It can be used safely by diabetics and people who are overweight.

It is selectively used by beneficial intestinal organisms, especially bifidobacteria in the large intestines. (*Leaky Gut* . . . , 2004)

Probiotics (promotes life) play a distinctive role in the symbiosis of the intestinal flora. They help keep the microbial balance in the intestinal tract. The term "probiotic" was defined as "organisms and substances which control the intestinal microbial balance."

It behooves us know the common probiotics that will help insure intestinal health. Some of these are Lactobacillus acidophilus, and Bifidobacterium bifidus available in some yogurts and kefir. It pays to practice reading labels. Do not assume that these probiotics are present in the yogurt you buy unless "active cultures" is explicitly stated on the label.

Just What Do the Probiotics Do?

Dr. Harry K. Panjwani, M.D., Ph.D. has written the following discourse on probiotics, entitled "Just What Do the Probiotics Do?" reprinted here with permission:

It must be stressed that in the human gastrointestinal tract where not only absorption of food takes place but also our immune systems and other protection mechanisms are also maintained. Natural microflora—approximately 400 different types of living bacterial micro-organisms—establish themselves in the intestinal tract. They help the body fight infections. They are affected adversely by improper diet, such as excessive use of refined foods, long-term use of antibiotics and other medications, stressful lifestyle, and bad habits.

In recent years, we have had a proliferation of coffee houses, cyber cafes, cigar clubs, in spite of what we know about damage from excessive use of nicotine, sugar, and caffeine. The human body is a very well designed intricate piece of machinery which should be kept in balance and well maintained. Add to that family disruptions, job and financial problems, long work hours, hasty meals, long commutes, hard to handle pollution of air soil and water, and a lack of adequate sleep and water intake. They all work against us.

Probiotics are the intestinal flora, notably lactobacillus acidophilus (present in the small intestine) and bifodobacterium bifidus (present in the colon). Intestinal flora are made up of many kinds of living bacteria which maintain a symbiotic relationship with the rest of the body. L. acidophilus and B. bifidus are available as supplements, not unlike vitamins and minerals when the body may be deficient. They are gatekeepers of the body and help with absorption of the nutrients and elimination of pathogens and toxins. For example, bloating and gas formation are common uncomfortable symptoms when probiotics are deficient. Yogurt has been used for centuries as a source of probiotics. It is particularly helpful in lactose intolerant persons. Lactic ferments in yogurt secrete enzymes like lactase that convert lactose into lactic acid. They make lactose more digestible.

Probiotics also promote absorption of calcium and provide B vitamins.

They are helpful in the elderly where it helps with constipation by promoting intestinal peristalsis and lowering pH. They especially play an important role in combating infections, lowered resistance, tiredness and dull skin. They maintain a balance between different micro-organisms in the intestinal tract, most of which are usually harmless. They also inhibit pathogenic bacteria. Antibiotics, especially prolonged use, and also indirectly through use of meat products fed to cattle, results in overproduction of Candida (fungus) and can be controlled with probiotics.

We do not yet know what impact genetically modified foods may have since such foods do not always carry the necessary label and are not being monitored yet. Cheese, miso and tempeh are also helpful but do not provide long term colonization of the intestine, whereas the use of supplements is more consistent. Their ability to create low acidic pH, especially in the intestine and vagina, does not allow the growth of pathogenic bacteria. Other possible uses of probiotics are in irritable bowel syndrome, yeast infections, lactose intolerance (partial or complete), urinary tract infection, and may reduce the risk of colon cancer and is known to lower cholesterol. It is helpful in post-cancer patients on chemotherapy or radiation where diarrhea is common which may be relieved by probiotics.

Like most medical and nutritional products, it is available in tablet, powder, liquid and capsule form and can also be used as a vaginal douche. It is always prudent that any treatment should be medically supervised as a cautionary measure. Probiotics are considered safe and have no known side effects, no toxicity or contraindications. They are adversely affected by alcohol, excessive use of antibiotics and prevent recurrent infections after intermittent use of antibiotics. Probiotics are commonly used in Europe, in conjunction with appropriate diet.   (Harry K. Panjwani, M.D., Ph.D.)

Lactobacillus acidophilus helps prevent pathogenic bacteria from proliferating and healthy bacteria from becoming toxic. This is well documented. As stated earlier, bifidobacteria is also a probiotic found primarily in the large intestine. When Candida albicans developed in an infant after being treated with penicillin therapy, they orally administered a bifidus milk preparation for seven days. At the end of that period, there was a significant *increase* in the population of bifidobacteria and a *decrease* in the growth of Candida albicans, as observed in the feces.

The most practical probiotic on the market is plain yogurt with no fruit and no fat. Remember, the label should read "active cultures." This is also available in capsule form.

Goat's Milk

When it comes to allergens, milk in its present form can have a decided adverse effect on children and adults, especially if they suffer from eczema. In such cases, I place my very young patients on soy or goat's milk. Some can be allergic to soy milk and soy products, so I prefer goat's milk for the following reasons. Goat's milk:

- Is less allergenic than cow's milk.
- Does not suppress the immune system.
- Is easier to digest than cow's milk.
- Has more acid–buffering capacity.
- Alkalizes the digestive system. It produces an alkaline ash and does not produce acid in the system.
- Helps to increase the pH of the blood because it is the dairy product highest in the amino acid, L–glutamine, which is an alkaline form–

ing amino acid. If you recall, L-glutamine is one of the most powerful substances that helps repair a damaged intestinal wall.

* Does not produce mucus.
* Does not stimulate a defense response from the immune system.

Dietary Fiber

Dietary fiber as a supportive substance to a probiotic is another such aid that exerts a beneficial effect on human health by improving the balance of the intestinal flora.

An interesting study with laboratory animals showed that adding fiber (cellulose powder) to a liquid diet *decreased* the ability for bacteria to translocate, that is, pass through the intestinal barrier due to a leaky gut. "Thus the oral administration of this fiber maintains intestinal barrier function and prevents bacterial translocation even in the absence of oral nutrients." (Percival, 1999, p. 4)

There are many formulas on the market today that are effective fiber products. To name a few: psyllium husks, Fibercon, and Metamucil. Remember, however, when fiber supplements are used, it is essential to drink plenty of water since fiber expands when ingested.

In one test, a high cholesterol diet was fed to eight adult individuals without any fiber. To another group, a high cholesterol diet again was given, but this time they added 15 grams of fiber. The addition of the fiber was noteworthy when the final results were in.

Mitsuoka, a researcher, commented on the study once the findings were compiled: "These results suggest that the high cholesterol diet increased putrefying bacteria and putrefactive products. Dietary fiber (on the other hand) exerts a beneficial effect on human health by improving the balance of the intestinal flora." (Percival, 1999, p. 4)

13

The Healing Crisis

Experiencing the Herxheimer Reaction

Whether you call it the healing crisis, the purge period, the terrible time, or any other similar name, the fact is that once the normal immune system starts to kick in the body goes through a cleansing period in which every pore of the skin surface becomes inflamed, dry, sore, and, in general, puts the patient through a living hell! While this does not happen to everyone, to those who do experience it, all I can say is "Hang in there. Relief is on the way!" It is the body purging itself.

No matter how I emphasize this to a new patient and assure them that even though the condition they come in with will worsen as the body's defense system starts throwing off all the accumulated toxins, there are some who, once it starts to happen, simply can't handle it.

In scientific terms it is referred to as the Herxheimer or "die-off" reaction. This occurs not only in psoriasis and eczema cases but even more frequently in cases of yeast overgrowth. The trick is to get through this inflammatory period in any way possible while the healing is taking place throughout the body cells.

I recall one severely afflicted patient of mine who was going through this period, who, when I called to ask her how she was doing, replied, "Oh, I'm doing great—I'm flared-up all over!" It wasn't long before the reaction reached its peak and she began to sense the relief. Her skin surface no longer itched, the dryness subsided, blotched areas of light skin began to break through, and she "knew" she was getting better. It was only a couple of weeks later that she experienced a total skin renewal without a blemish on it.

A photographic sequence of a severe Herxheimer reaction that took place on one of my male patients is shown in the color photographic section of this book. This patient only had to go to his medical doctor once for a diuretic when swelling up of his lower legs occurred. It was resolved in a few days and the patient continued with the cleansing regimen to a successful outcome.

When yeast overgrowth is the primary culprit, this "die-off" period comes through loud and clear. "This means that so many yeasts die that their chemical by-products, of which there are 180, flood the system and make a person's symptoms feel worse," as reported by Carolyn Dean, M.D., N.D., Medical Health Advisor, Yeast Connection.Com. I urge anyone suffering from yeast infestation to check Dr. Dean's site at www.yeastconnection.com/fighting_ask.html and find out about her "yeast fighting program."

For a 2–3 week period, Dr. Dean emphasizes the avoidance of all fruit (because of its fruit sugar [fructose] content), as well as sugar, alcohol, processed foods, yeast, and yeast–laden foods and fungi. By avoiding such food items, symptoms of yeast overgrowth will significantly be reduced. More information may be obtained by visiting her Web site listed above.

In my experience, the greatest aid a patient experiencing the Herxheimer Reaction can give himself is the following:

1. Drink plenty of fresh water—perhaps 10 glasses of pure water a day.

2. A home enema, perhaps one a day for the first three days once the crisis begins.

3. A tepid bath followed by a good moisturizer such as Hydrophilic Ointment or Aveeno Deep moisturizer.

4. A high colonic irrigation in severe cases, perhaps once or twice a week until the crisis passes. (Drinking plenty of water will help to prevent dehydration.)

5. A high alkaline diet, particularly green leafy vegetables, but no fruit for the time being even though most of them are alkaline reacting in the body (Note: an effective homemade vegetable drink is the juicing of romaine lettuce, celery, and a tablespoon each of watercress and parsley to which a tablespoon of olive oil is added after it is processed.)

6. Plain yogurt and acidophilus.

7. Garlic Health Boat (see recipe given earlier): One or two of these is suggested daily unless the patient has an underlying gastritis or ulcer that may cause discomfort. This is a tasty way to get the two most effective natural ingredients, garlic and olive oil, to the walls of the intestines, where the folds harbor the yeast microorganism and help neutralize and flush it out.

Undoubtedly, there are prescription medications, namely Nystatin and Diflucan, among others, and herbal supplements that claim to do the same thing, but since I do not deal with such items, I recommend that my patients who are interested in these things consult with their medical practitioner for the latest recommendation on the allopathic approach to the disease.

The main thing to grasp in this section of the discussion is to realize that the *Herxheimer Reaction is the body's attempt to help you.* To help it along and speed up the recovery time is the purpose of this chapter. As far as how long it will take to detox is anybody's guess. I have seen it happen in a few days to a few weeks. I always refer to it as the most difficult ordeal of the entire healing process for both the patient and doctor.

Regardless of what measures are taken to heal a leaky gut, they are practically worthless if the patient does not include the elements of *time* and *patience,* as well as *faith.*

Remember, it took time to get sick—consequently, it will take time to get well! Give it a chance to work is my advice to every one of my patients. I tell them to be grateful for little signs of healing as they occur. Those little signs mean the protocol is working. Now, the trick is to follow through.

I remind them that even during flare-up periods they should be persistent until the crisis passes. That's all part of the healing process. Admittedly, it is the most difficult time, but with understanding of what is happening (the body is being purified of toxins), with time and patience the changes will come and the healing will have a better chance of taking place. I have seen this happen time and time again.

However, in all honesty, this "purge" period could last a long time, perhaps months. This "die off" period can be most discouraging. It takes a great deal of faith and encouragement from the loved ones surrounding the patient. The only thing one can do during the healing crisis is to keep flushing the system out by drinking plenty of fresh water. The idea is to prevent the toxins, whatever they may be, from building up again and watch for little signs of improvement. *It is extremely difficult to convince a patient that this purge period is actually a blessing.* Always keep in mind to check with your personal physician as to your general state of health during this "terrible time."

As part of the healing process I urge my patients to surround themselves with people of a constructive and positive nature—and avoid those who discourage them. Most, if not all, of those "close" acquaintances haven't a clue as to what is going on—and worse, they don't care enough to find out before they infect the patient with their discouraging words. The patient who is plagued with such acquaintances should retreat to a hidden chamber within and put up a sign reading "No admittance" when in the presence of such people.

As much as I stress that the patient should avoid certain foods that have proven to be toxic to the body, I look the same way upon the influence of mental toxins that can be just as destructive as a diet that is poison to the body. With a view to not allowing such influences to take hold in the mental economy of the patient, I recommend the patient get rid of such thoughts by taking a mental "enema" just as I would suggest a physical enema to help rid the body of accumulated toxins. Just as healing thoughts are an energy that flows through every portion of our being, destructive thoughts do likewise. The energy will flow through us, and the form it takes will be determined by our thoughts. It is manifested in the physical structures and processes of our bodies and the behavior patterns of our lives.

We cannot see thought—no more than we can see electricity or the wind, but we can certainly perceive the effects of such. That is why modern psychologists agree with Cayce, who suggested: "Keep the constructive mental attitude." (281-54) This applies to every aspect of life.

Unwanted "Help"

One factor that doesn't help the patient or the doctor is when people close to the patient see what they are going through and spread their fear and concern to the patient. Usually they did not attend the early consultations when all of this was explained to the patient. They only see the crisis in full blown form, and they panic. To say this is frustrating is to put it mildly! Although I can appreciate their concern for their loved one, they are of no help; in fact they are a detriment. Such people would do well to just disappear until the crisis is over. Then, as outspoken as they were during the crisis, they often remain mute, and you hardly hear from them again.

This may seem to my readers as a rough-and-ready mode of expression on my part, but my interest is focused on the patient, not on those around him. If they are not helping, they are a hindrance. It is a problem that I believe all physicians will face from time to time in their practice. My purpose in emphasizing this aspect of the healing process is, in some small way, to remind my readers, especially treating physicians, that "To be forewarned is to be forearmed."

Overweight

When one thinks about it, there is an answer to how understanding the leaky gut can lead to weight control.

Consider the following: One of the beneficial side effects I have witnessed in the healing of psoriasis and eczema is the loss of weight that occurs when following the dietary measures called for in both conditions. The high alkaline/low acidic diet in itself plays the major role because acidic foods are primarily proteins derived from meats and grains. Red meat is particularly avoided, thus curtailing cholesterol content and saturated fats. Sugar and sweets in general, are very restricted, as is the intake of junk food. These are all the foods that put on the extra baggage.

To illustrate: A patient came to me with one of the worst cases of psoriasis on record. Lesions covered practically every square inch of her body. The skin was thick, scaly, and stiff. She could hardly move without the pain of cracking and splitting skin. To add to her dilemma, she weighed in at 250 pounds!

For twenty-eight years she was treated at one of the leading psoriasis university centers in the country, and believe it or not, by the same physician who was also the head of the dermatology department. She was constantly seeking answers, for the results obtained at the psoriasis center left much to be desired. My book, *Healing Psoriasis: The Natural Alternative*, was given to her by a friend. She expressed her joy when she said, "The minute I saw the cover, I knew this was going to help me!"

It was not an easy task, for, not only were the dietary changes a difficult discipline for her, but the flare-up periods, of which there were three during the healing phase, put her through the pain of hell—but she stayed with it! Besides that, she had to drive two hours to my office for each visit. In spite of that, she agreed to come to my office once a week until she cleared. It took two years to accomplish, but at that time she appeared as living proof of the efficacy of this alternative approach to the disease, and, as an added benefit, she lost 100 pounds!

When I addressed a packed audience at the Fort Lee Historic Park Museum in Fort Lee, New Jersey, this patient agreed to appear as a living witness to a successful outcome. To say that she was an inspiration to everyone in the audience is to put it mildly.

A few weeks after this, the ever-popular television program, *60 Minutes*, contacted me and requested an interview for a possible TV special. Of course I agreed, as did this patient and three others. Two producers of *60 Minutes* came to my office and saw and heard the stories of each patient. They were so impressed that as they left the office they turned to me and said, "We think we have the story of the year. We will go back to our main office (in New York) with our highest recommendation."

I never heard from them again. After a few months, I thought I would check up on the status of our meeting so I called the station. The project had been turned over to another producer, one who did not share the enthusiasm of the producers who took the time to meet the patients personally. The project was discarded and forgotten, but not before I learned that the studio had called the doctor who had been treating her for 28 years and asked him what he thought of my approach to the disease, especially in the light of the results obtained. His answer, as reported to me, was, "Dr. Pagano is doing everything wrong. But his patients are getting well." Now you figure that one out!

The long and short of this story is that by following the regimen based on the leaky gut, the patient responded far beyond her fondest expectations and in the meantime lost 100 pounds! So, loss of weight is frequently a benefit welcomed by the patient. There have been times, however, when a patient may lose too much weight. That is usually easily corrected by having them double up on the permitted foods. The amount of food ingested does not seem to be as significant as the *selection* of foods.

Maintaining the pH Balance

Of all the various processes that go on in the human body for the maintenance of good health, none is more important than the maintaining of a normal acid/base balance. This means that fluids that make up every cell of your body should tend slightly towards the alkaline (base) side rather than the acidic. The body humors (fluids) are measured by what is called pH. The term "pH" stands for protein bound hydrogen. The neutral reading is based on the pH of water which is 7. Any reading below that number indicates acidity; any reading above that number signifies alkalinity. The body maintains a proper state of health when the blood registers 7.365; in other words, just a little above 7.0. Even a small percentage above that point could spell trouble. Depending upon the extent of acids in the body, anything below the figure of 7.0 indicates the amount of acidity in the blood.

Why is this important? Because too much acidity breaks down the barrier wall of the intestines, feeds the yeast, fungus, and molds that gather in the convolutions of the small intestine and nourishes the germs, bacteria, parasites and microforms proliferating their growth and resistance.

What is it that primarily promotes or prevents acidity? You might have guessed it—*your daily diet!* Make no mistake about it. It is what you put in your mouth that determines what comes out through your skin, what locks up your joints, what makes your muscles ache and what causes your depression. Emotions and environmental factors also play a part.

Dr. Robert Young, M.D., author of *The pH Miracle*, and world-renowned authority on pH and its influence in general health has this to say:

> Microacidity and microform overgrowth are inextricably linked. Microforms are a major source of acid in the body. Acidification creates a comfy environment for microforms. We predispose ourselves to both conditions through various stresses. The main one is poor diet . . .

He continues:

> First comes something that disturbs your body in some way, be it poor diet, polluted environment, negative thoughts, spiritual distress, or destructive emotions. Whatever it may be, that initial physical or emotional disturbance starts acidifying your body and disturbs your very cells. Cells work to adapt to the declining pH of their compromised environment. They break down and evolve to bacteria, yeast, fungus and molds. These in turn create their waste products—debilitating acids—which further pollute the environment. That in itself is a disturbance to the system, and in this way the whole cycle keeps rolling along. (Young, 2002)

Testing Your pH

There are immediate home testing devices that can give you an idea of your body's pH—pH of 7 is considered to be the neutral base line. Any number below 7 indicates acidity and the lower the number, the higher the amount of acidity. Anything above 7 reveals the amount of alkalinity in your body. Remember, the most desirable blood pH is 7.365. Your doctor can order this test for you. But litmus paper or pH strips that measure saliva or urine are available in a drug store or health food store. Its action is based on the color that appears after placing the strip of the litmus in your mouth and allowing the saliva to act on it for one or two seconds. The urine is tested by saturating the tip of the strip. In either case, you compare the resulting color with the color code on the dispenser to determine your reading. (The urine is best tested first thing in the morning.)

You want the middle of the road, that is, if the strip turns too dark or blue, it is too basic or alkaline, if it is too light or yellow it is too acidic. The ideal is to have the color be a medium green. There are also battery–operated pH electron meters which are accurate but can be expensive. For more on pH testing, refer to Dr. Young's most informative book *The pH Miracle.*

Even the highly respected Andrew Weil, M.D., acknowledges the importance of pH. Jerry Shaw provides the following quote from Dr. Weil where he was speaking of thrush, an infection of the mouth and throat. "Since Candida is always living in our guts in the yeast form, we just don't want it to overgrow or to morph [change] into the fungal form. **Maintaining proper intestinal pH is key to maintaining a healthy body.''** (emphasis added) (Shaw)

14

---•-•—•—•-•—•-•—•-•—

Psoriasis and Eczema

There are two reasons why I have chosen to close this work with psoriasis and eczema as they relate to leaky gut syndrome:

1. They both have as their etiology the same gut origin; namely intestinal permeability or leaky gut, in most cases. In some cases, the patient may have a combination of the two conditions.

2. They both require the same approach to their alleviation: a high alkaline diet, the use of the same herb teas (slippery elm bark powder and American yellow saffron tea (except in cases of pregnancy).

All other natural measures that I have incorporated in the management of both conditions are virtually the same: clean out the system with plenty of water, natural cathartics, colonic irrigation (in severe cases) and plenty of green leafy vegetables. If yeast overgrowth is suspected, encourage the use of probiotics (lactobacillus and bifidobacterium species), olive oil, and fresh garlic. Be sure there is no constipation problem. A bowel movement *one to three times a day is normal for everyone* (not only once or twice a week!).

The use of topical oils is generally the same: a good moisturizer combined with an olive oil/peanut oil mixture (50-50) is most popular. Spi-

133

nal adjustments also have a positive role to play.

Then, the importance of time and patience: allow time for it to happen. In both cases, there may be a yeast "die off" period that could be a living hell for the patient (the Herxheimer Reaction). There may be more than one episode before it all begins to calm down. Once that happens, at least with those that I have treated, improvement continues to a final successful outcome.

Can the condition return? Yes, it certainly can if the patient prematurely reverts to the eating habits that brought on the condition in the first place. In one case of mine, however, it was seventeen years before psoriasis began to raise its head again. The patient simply got back on the diet and soon he was in control again!

Probably one of the most rewarding aspects of healing both psoriasis and/or eczema in this manner is that in practically every case I had, the patient never feared the disease again! If a patient broke out again, the patient could often trace it quickly to a violation of the regimen. The patient knew why the outbreak had occurred and could get right back on track. The difference now was that the patient had a choice and was largely in control of the condition. To me this is almost as gratifying as clearing up the problem itself.

Psoriasis and/or Eczema in Young Children

In my experience, children, from toddler age to mid–teens, clear up faster than adults. The average young person can clear up in anywhere from one to three months. In two cases, both five–year–olds, it only took two weeks! Most of these children were on junk food. All those sweets, sodas, candy, and sugar products of every description in general were the basic underlying cause. As I have mentioned quite clearly in earlier sections of this book, in many cases, *it is what the patient stays away from that brings about a healing.*

The best results come about in families where the parents take charge of children's eating habits. They are told what they can have and what they cannot have. When they see and experience the improvement, they would not break the rules. The children look better, feel better, and most of all, they are free of pain and disfigurement.

In the Case of Newborns

Yes, a child can actually be born with psoriasis or eczema lesions. You may ask how that can be. The baby didn't have time to pollute himself. So the question is where did the toxins come from? Where else but from the mother! That's why the mother should still follow the basic rules of 80%–20% alkaline/acid diet during the gestation period. Of course there are always exceptions—that's why a woman should always check with her obstetrician before embarking on any dietary plan during pregnancy. It is also advisable to avoid slippery elm and saffron tea during this time. Such incidences, lesions of the newborn, have taken place while the baby is being breast-fed. My suggestion has always been that the nursing mother should check with her obstetrician for approval, and, if given, she should follow the basis rules of the diet herself. The transfer of toxins from the mother to the infant will stop and the baby responds accordingly.

If I have done anything in my nearly half century of clinical practice, it has been to prove that, in most cases, a patient with psoriasis or eczema does not necessarily have to live with either of these debilitating diseases! The question is whether the patient is willing to pay the price. That price is not measured in dollars and cents, but in time, patience and discipline. To repeat the most valuable words of Edgar Cayce, to all psoriasis (and eczema) patients the world over, regarding a cure for these maladies:

> **Most of this is found in *diet*. There is a cure. It requires patience, persistence, and right thinking also!**   2455-2

In my opinion this bit of advice applies equally well in cases of leaky gut syndrome.

15

Using Our Mental Powers

The Law of Expectancy

I end this work with a few thoughts on a subject which few practitioners would routinely consider to have anything to do with the healing of disease—that of the *attitude* of both the patient and the doctor!

Perhaps one of the earliest accounts of the effect the mind has on the relief, alleviation and healing of a disease condition in the modern world was described by Thompson J. Hudson as long ago as 1903 in his classic work *The Law of Mental Medicine*. In his account he cited an experiment that proved to be quite profound regarding the effect mental attitude has on a person's well being.

A number of patients with the same problem were divided into two groups. One group was given a medication accompanied by an explanation of its purpose. The second group was administered the same medication without any indication of what it was supposed to accomplish. After a determined amount of time, the patients in both groups were reevaluated with striking results. The group that received the medication and the explanation responded quite well, whereas the group who had received only the medication and no explanation of what to expect remained the same or even got worse! Yes, that was over a hundred years ago, but, I would expect a similar experiment conducted today to yield the same results. How often have we heard stories about how a person did not know something was impossible, so he went ahead and did it!

See It—Believe It—Live It:
The Art of Visualization

All the therapeutic measures up to this point deal with physical applications, dietary measures, lifestyle changes, etc. But there is another dimension that, I daresay, may be most rewarding to anyone with a physical or mental problem in need of correction—the *art of visualization*.

By that is meant, in its simplest terms, see (in your mind's eye) the problem as being solved, the therapeutic suggestions as working, the gut wall as being healed over, and your state of health restored. This is an area that has seldom been recognized, much less taught, in medical institutions or health facilities. This reverts back to the Law of Expectancy. It carries with it the Wisdom of the Ages.

For instance, see the L. Acidophilus or yogurt replacing the acidifying bacteria by overwhelming numbers, thereby rendering them ineffective. See the garlic and olive oil destroying the yeast microforms which will allow the friendly bacteria to grow and protect the intestinal walls.

Has this been proven, you may ask? Can the mind truly affect the gut interior wall? Let the researchers at Tufts University answer. This excerpt is taken from a feature article titled "Hypnosis for the Gut" and sheds some light on this question.

> A recent study suggests that hypnotherapy may provide relief to people suffering from what health professionals call recurrent upper-abdominal discomfort—but what you know as chronic indigestion . . .
>
> Researchers in England assigned 126 patients to one of three treatments for 4 months. One group took ranitidine (Zantac), a drug that reduces the amount of acid produced by the stomach. Another group received emotional support.

They also took a placebo pill that they were told could reduce stomach acid. The third group underwent hypnotherapy, which used relaxation, suggestion, and visualization to help people imagine their symptoms improving.

The people who received hypnotherapy reported the greatest improvement in symptoms. In addition, nearly three-quarters of the hypnosis group continued to feel better 10 months later, as opposed to just 43 percent in the drug group and 34 percent of those who received supportive therapy. Moreover, no one who received hypnotherapy sought out medication during the 10-month follow-up period, while the majority of people in the other treatment groups did.

(Tufts, August 2003)

Thus, the effect the mind has on the intestinal tract *if put into practice!* So, rather than exhaust your brain trying to figure out the reason that such knowledge is rarely brought to our attention, let's just get on with it! Realize it does help in many cases and helps us put into motion the most powerful force on earth that the human being is heir to—the Power of the Mind!

In other words, your mental attitude can and does play a decided role in the healing of disease as it does in any human endeavor. In today's world, such pioneers as Deepak Chopra and Larry Dorsey help blaze a trail to this profound concept. What remains really is the patient's awareness of his own powers of perception. For the most part, they do not exercise their mental powers because they are not aware of them.

More and more however this new concept in healing is gaining a foothold and programs, TV shows, radio personalities, news articles, books and magazines are endorsing such information, thereby lifting the veil of secrecy and coming forth with information, with the public clamoring for more.

The first group mentioned in Hudson's experiment were told the reason behind the medication, thus their mind focused on what to *expect*. The second, uninformed, group, did not know one way or the other what to expect, so nothing happened. The lesson of this story is simply that "You get what you think about."

So, if we get what we think about, why not expect the best for our–

selves as well as others? Every great philosopher declared it, every great military leader, from Alexander to Napoleon to Patton, more often than not has proved it.

That is why I emphasize having the right attitude, one of expectancy, when I lecture and give personal interviews on patients suffering from a condition that has origins in a leaky gut. I show them evidence of healing, before and after photos, have patients meet with other success-ful patients, have them contact each other (always with their permis-sion of course)—all with one goal in mind—that they can *expect* to be healed. The key is that I give them reason to believe it!

After you have added to your arsenal of remedies, an expectant men-tal attitude can be your most potent weapon, which in fact, can create miracles.

Throughout the Edgar Cayce discourses we find repeated references to guard our thoughts, not to allow what I call mental toxins to enter our spiritual environment any more than we would allow physical tox-ins to enter our bodies—or at least not to retain them! Cayce put it most succinctly in reading 456-1 when he said:

> Do all with that expectancy of that which is desired to be accomplished in this body and it will come to pass.

Truly a profound statement from which we may all benefit!

Appendix

A Man Named Edgar Cayce

In the summer of 1902 a little girl named Aime Dietrich was diagnosed as having a progressive brain disease with no hope for recovery. It was simply a matter of time before five-year-old Aime would succumb to this affliction which seemed to have started at the age of two when, according to her mother, she caught "the grippe." After the condition seemed to have run its course, she began to fall down suddenly; her body would stiffen and become rigid; signs of mental retardation were apparent. She was examined and treated for two years, but the condition worsened to the point of her having as many as twenty convulsions a day. Her mind stopped developing. Her devoted parents, having exhausted all avenues of hope, resigned themselves to the unbearable task of waiting for the end. They brought her home to die.

It was at this time that, through a neighbor, they heard of a young man named Edgar Cayce who, it was claimed, had a very unusual ability to diagnose and prescribe curative suggestions to those suffering from various ailments by placing himself in a trance-like state. In desperation, the Dietrichs, having no place else to turn, requested a "reading" from the young man. The humble, obliging Cayce agreed to try to help. As he had done many times before, even at this early stage of his calling, he unfastened his tie, loosened his shoelaces, reclined on his couch and began to relax. At that particular reading, it was Mr. Al C. Layne who conducted the session (others had conducted previous readings). Mr. Layne was later to become a graduate osteopath who not only conducted the hypnotic sessions, but also followed through on treatments of the patient if osteopathic therapy was required.

In a procedure that was to become a familiar pattern, Cayce apparently went to sleep. Then Mr. Layne began to speak, telling him that before him was the body of the child. He was to examine her and reveal the cause and cure of her condition.

In a few moments the "sleeping" Cayce began to speak in a very different, authoritative voice. "Yes, we have the body." He continued to relate that the day before Aime caught the grippe she suffered an injury to a segment of her spine. The grippe germs then settled in this area and became the focal point of infection that in turn affected the central nervous system. He advised specific spinal adjustments of an osteopathic nature.

After two attempts at adjusting the spine failed, subsequent readings insisted that the adjustments be performed in a very specific manner. This time, Mr. Layne followed directions explicitly and results were seen within a week. Aime's mind began to clear. Mr. Layne continued the treatments every day for three weeks and the child recovered completely. Aime's mother recalled that the day before she caught the grippe, Aime did, in fact, slip from a carriage step and injure the end of her spine. As the little girl didn't complain, her mother thought nothing of it. Three years after the incident, Aime's mind gradually began to develop normally once again after having received the therapeutic treatment suggested by Cayce.

Thus, another remarkable incident, early in his career, added to the legacy of Edgar Cayce; an incredible, amazing story that continues to startle the scientific community by offering causes and therapy for the most baffling diseases.

The range of treatments called for in the readings for specific individuals varied widely from spinal manipulation (of an osteopathic or chiropractic nature); to physiotherapy (which included massage and specific exercise); to hydrotherapy (baths and colonic irrigations); and with great emphasis on diet and dietary measures. There were several occasions where immediate surgery was recommended or specific drugs, some of which were so new on the market that the patient's physician was not aware of them.

One reading for a physical ailment required that the patient obtain a preparation called "Oil of Smoke." Dr. Wesley H. Ketchum, a young physician at the time who conducted this particular reading, had never heard of such a substance, nor had the local druggist. It was not even listed in the pharmaceutical catalogues. The reading then said it could be found in a drug store in Louisville. Dr. Ketchum wired the store asking for the preparation. The response from the store manager was that he did not have it nor had he ever heard of it. Another reading was given for clarification. This time Cayce in his trancelike state advised that not only did that particular store have it but directed the manager to look in the back of his drug store on a certain shelf. There behind another preparation he would find an old bottle of "Oil of Smoke." This was carried out. Much to everyone's delight and amazement, there stood a bottle of "Oil of Smoke."

Another documented account in the early life of Cayce was the case of Mr. P.A. Andrews of New York. While in his state of trance, Cayce diagnosed the man's condition, even though he was hundreds of miles away, and recommended a mixture known as Clarawater. No one, physicians included, knew of the existence of such a compound. When it became obvious that it was unobtainable, Mr. Andrews wrote to Cayce informing him of the situation and that he had even advertised for it in various medical journals, to no avail. He requested another reading in which perhaps Cayce could give the specific formula which could then be made up by a pharmacist. Cayce agreed, went into a trance, and came forth with the specific ingredients and formula for Clarawater. Mr. Andrews followed through and began to feel better after taking it.

It was not too long before Edgar received a letter from Mr. Andrews. He had related to Cayce that he received a letter from a man in Paris, France, who had seen his advertisement for Clarawater. He went on to inform him that he is quite aware of it, since it was his father who had invented it. Although it was no longer available, he took it upon himself to at least send the formula to Mr. Andrews. When he compared the dosages and ingredients, it was found to be exactly, in every detail, the same formula brought forth by Cayce.

Such incidents abound in the forty–three years in which Cayce gave readings. The reading did not single out any particular health field as being more valuable than another. The best therapy was the therapy that would get the job done. This is adequately expressed in a reading given in 1939:

> Know that all strength, all healing of every nature is the changing of the vibrations from within—the attuning of the divine within the living tissue of a body to Creative Energies. This alone is healing. Whether it is accomplished by the use of drugs, the knife or what not, it is the attuning of the atomic structure of the living cellular force to its spiritual heritage.
> 1967-1

The story of Edgar Cayce has an origin as beautiful as the stories and case histories of the thousands of people helped by this remarkable man. It begins within the consciousness Edgar himself. As a very young man he had a deep appreciation for the Bible and read it fervently once a year for every year of his life. Normal school subjects took a back seat. Consequently, his grades suffered, for which his father, the Squire Cayce, brought the house down around him! However, his mother recognized her son's sensitivity, knowing intuitively he would one day be an honor to his family and community.

At the age of thirteen, he experienced what today would be referred to as an apparition. On a beautiful May afternoon in the woods, at his favorite spot for reading the Bible, he began to read the story of Manoah. Suddenly, he felt a presence, as if someone was standing nearby observing him. He looked up and saw in the rays of the sun the image of a woman. At first he thought it was his mother but soon realized it was someone strange to him. She spoke to him in a soft, musical voice. "Your prayers have been heard," she said. "Tell me what you would like most of all, so that I may give it to you."

Startled, he was wondering what had happened to him. She waited smilingly. He replied, "Most of all I would like to be helpful to others, especially to children when they are sick." Without a word, she disappeared.

He picked up his Bible and ran as fast as he could to tell his mother, "Do you think I've been reading the Bible too much?" He added, "It makes some people go crazy, doesn't it?" His mother assured him his prayers were answered and not to allow the incident to frighten him but to look upon it as a special message, even though at the moment it was not understood. She did advise, however, to keep it a secret.

The next day at school the daydreamer was higher in the clouds than usual. His spelling lesson turned out to be a disaster. He was sent home in disgrace. His father was determined to teach him a lesson, figuratively and literally. He pounded the lesson over and over into his son, without success. On three occasions, in total frustration, he slapped him to the floor. As he sat dejectedly, Edgar heard a voice within him, "If you can sleep a little, we can help you." He felt sure it was the voice of the beautiful woman he had met the day before.

Edgar convinced his father to allow him to rest on the book awhile. Reluctantly, his father permitted him to do so. Cayce went to sleep on the book immediately. When the squire returned, he snatched it from under his head, waking Edgar suddenly. "Ask me the lesson. I know it now," Edgar said.

The squire began. The answers were correct in every detail. When the boy asked his father to ask even the next day's lesson, he did so. Again all the answers were correct. This ability was to follow him through school—he would sleep on his lessons and know the answers, word for word, on awakening.

This marked the beginning of a power strange enough to stir his immediate friends and family, his community, and eventually, a nation. As the years passed, the extent of his ability became apparent when he was able to place himself in an altered state of consciousness, diagnose illnesses of individual people, and recommend remedies. This gift soon became known to the scientific community. It was on October 9, 1910, that the *New York Times* carried a full page display in its magazine section. The headline read, "Illiterate Man Becomes Doctor When Hypno-

tized—Strange Power Shown by Edgar Cayce Puzzles Physicians." The
first paragraph read:

> The medical fraternity of the country is taking a lively interest
> in the strange power said to be possessed by Edgar Cayce, of
> Hopkinsville, Kentucky, to diagnose difficult diseases while in
> a semi-conscious state, though he has not the slightest knowl-
> edge of medicine when not in this condition.

With an impressive track record already behind him, the question
most frequently asked was, "To what power or force do you and your
associates attribute this phenomenon?" The answer was printed in the
same New York Times story. While in the familiar state of trance, Cayce
spoke:

> Edgar Cayce's mind is amenable to suggestion, the same as
> all other subconscious minds, but in addition thereto it has
> the power to interpret to the objective mind of others what it
> acquired from the subconscious state of other individuals of
> the same kind. The subconscious mind forgets nothing. The
> conscious mind received the impression from without and
> transfers all thought to the subconscious, where it remains
> even though the conscious be destroyed.

Thus began what was to be the saga of Edgar Cayce—a saga that
became a living legend and in turn a legacy for the aid of humanity.

Little Aime Dietrich, for instance, was only one of over six thousand
persons whom Cayce helped through the years. These six thousand or
more cases provided over 14,000 readings on a multitude of diseases
ranging from the simple cold remedy to facts and suggestions on cancer; from a nerve impingement to multiple sclerosis, and from painful
joints to crippling arthritis. It is a matter of record that his diagnoses
and accuracy were determined at over 90 percent, a record enviable
and unmatched even in today's modern therapeutic managements.

Of the more than fourteen thousand readings now indexed and
housed in the library at the Association for Research and Enlightenment (A.R.E.) and Edgar Cayce Foundation headquarters in Virginia
Beach, some ten thousand are directly involved with matters of health

and well being. Physicians, therapists, educators and other members of the health fields are particularly invited to examine the records to reach their own conclusions as to their efficacy. The remaining discourses are divided among such subjects as geological heritage and changes in the earth, reincarnation, dreams and their meanings, planetary influences, attitudes and emotions, Atlantis, accounts of the Christ, and changes that may occur and are occurring in the earth today.

It was Edgar Cayce himself who had the strongest doubts about this strange, unorthodox method of advising and suggesting remedies for such a disparity of diseases. He made a vow early in his life as a psychic diagnostician that if even one person was harmed or made worse by following the suggestions, he would stop the readings and never again give another. For forty-three years, Cayce carried on his work almost to the very day of his death on January 3, 1945, with apparently no one ever being harmed or hurt by the suggestions.

References for Citations

Abel, Robert, Jr., M.D. (1999) *The Eye Care Revolution* New York: Kensington Health Books.

AIA Newsletter No. 18 (Summer 1997) What Is Leaky Gut Syndrome? Retrieved from osiris.sunderland.ac.uk/autism/gut.htm on March 18, 2006.

Ball, Eddy, Runkel, Patrick, and Holmes, Scott (Eds.). (1999) *Functional Assessment Resource Manual*, Asheville, NC: Great Smokies Diagnostic Laboratory

Balch, James, F., M.D. and Balch, Phyllis, CNC (1997) *Prescription for Nutritional Healing* (2nd ed.). Garden City Park, NY: Avery Publishing Group.

Best and Taylor, (1955) *Physiological Basis of Medical Practice*, (6th ed.) Baltimore: Williams and Wilkins Company.

Bingham, Max (n.d.) *Autism and the Human Gut Flora*. Retrieved from osiris.sunderland.ac.uk/autism/gut.htm on 3/18/ 2006

Brady, Diane. (2006, October 16) The Organic Myth. *Business Week.*

Cabot, Sandra, M.D. (n.d.) *Leaky Gut Syndrome*. Retrieved on 3/18/2006 from www.liverdoctor.com/04_leakygut_syndrome.asp

Childers, Norman, F. (1989) *Nightshades Newsletter*

Chusid, Joseph G. and McDonald, Joseph G. (1954). *Correlative Neuroanatomy and Functional Neurology*. Los Altos, CA: Lange Medical Publications.

Clemente, Carmine D. ed. (1985) *Gray's Anatomy* 30th ed., Philadelphia: Lea and Febiger

Cobb, Mark and Cobb, Alyson. (n.d.) *Eliminate the Underlying Cause*. Retrieved from www.Candidafree.net on 3/18/2006.

Crook, William G. M.D. (2000) *The Yeast Connection Handbook*. Jackson, TN: The Yeast Connection.

Dean, Carolyn, M.D., N.D. (n.d.) www.yeastconnection.com/fighting_ask.html

Gabbay, Simone (Sept./Oct. 1998) *Venture Inward*

Galland, Leo M.D., (n.d.) *Leaky Gut Syndromes: Breaking the Vicious Cycle*. Retrieved from www.mdheal.org/leakygut.htm on 3/18/2006

Hudson, Thompson J. (1903) *The Law of Mental Medicine*

Hunter, Beatrice T. (1987) *Gluten Intolerance* Keats Publishing

Karp, Reba Ann. (1986) *The Edgar Cayce Encyclopedia of Healing*, Warner Books, Inc.

Larson, David E., M.D., Editor-in-Chief (1990) *Mayo Clinic Family Healthbook*, William Morrow

Leaky Gut: The Diseases Have Different Names but One Thing in Common (July 2004), *ACCM Health Sense*, X,7, Irving, TX: The American Council on Collaborative Medicine, Inc.

McGarey, William A., M.D. (March 1979) Notes from the Medical Research Bulletin, A.R.E. Journal

McGarey, William A., M.D. (1994) Healing is Simple, Yet Magnificent *Venture Inward*

McGarey, William A., M.D. ( ) *The Oil that Heals*. Virginia Beach, VA: ARE Press

National Digestive Diseases Information Clearinghouse (NDDIC) (n.d.) *Celiac Disease*, Retrieved from digestive.niddk.nih.gov/ddiseases/pubs/celiac/#1 on March 18, 2006

Pagano, John O.A. (1991) *Healing Psoriasis: The Natural Alternative*. Englewood Cliifs, NJ: The Pagano Organization

Percival, Mark. (1999) *Intestinal Health*. Applied Nutritional Science Report. Vol. 15 No. 5

Physician's Reference Notebook. (1968) Virginia Beach, VA: A.R.E. Press

Rapaport, Lisa, Cortez, Michelle F., and Washburn, Linda. (Oct. 7, 2006) "J&J Drug OK'd for Symptoms of Autism" Hackensack, NJ: *The Record*

Reilly, Harold J. and Brod, Ruth H. (1975) *The Edgar Cayce Handbook for Health through Drugless Therapy*. New York: Macmillan Publishing Co., Inc.

Rubin, Jordan S. (2004-5) *The Maker's Diet*. Lake Mary, FL: Siloam

Shaw, Jerry. ( ) *The Healing Power of Olive Oil*. Boca Raton, FL: Globe Communications Corp.

Tufts University Health and Nutrition Letter (April 2003)

Tufts University Health and Nutrition Letter (August 2003) Hypnosis for the Gut.

Tufts University Health and Nutrition Letter (October 2006)

Washburn, Linda (Sept. 2006) "In Autism's Grip" Hackensack, NJ: *The Record*

Young, Robert, Ph.D., and Young, Shelly R. (2002) *The pH Miracle*. New York: Warner Books

A.R.E. PRESS

The A.R.E. Press publishes books, videos, audiotapes, CDs, and DVDs meant to improve the quality of our readers' lives—personally, professionally, and spiritually. We hope our products support your endeavors to realize your career potential, to enhance your relationships, to improve your health, and to encourage you to make the changes necessary to live a loving, joyful, and fulfilling life.

For more information or to receive a free catalog, call:

800–333–4499

Or write:

A.R.E. Press
215 67th Street
Virginia Beach, VA 23451-2061

ARE PRESS.COM

BAAR PRODUCTS

A.R.E.'s Official Worldwide Exclusive Supplier of Edgar Cayce Health Care Products

Baar Products, Inc., is the official worldwide exclusive supplier of Edgar Cayce health care products. Baar offers a collection of natural products and remedies drawn from the work of Edgar Cayce, considered by many to be the father of modern holistic medicine.

For a complete listing of Cayce-related products, call:

800–269–2502

Or write:

Baar Products, Inc.
P.O. Box 60
Downingtown, PA 19335 U.S.A.

Customer Service and International: 610-873-4591
Fax: 610-873-7945
Web Site: www.baar.com   E-mail: cayce@baar.com

EDGAR CAYCE'S A.R.E.

What Is A.R.E.?

The Association for Research and Enlightenment, Inc., (A.R.E.®) was founded in 1931 to research and make available information on psychic development, dreams, holistic health, meditation, and life after death. As an open–membership research organization, the A.R.E. continues to study and publish such information, to initiate research, and to promote conferences, distance learning, and regional events. Edgar Cayce, the most documented psychic of our time, was the moving force in the establishment of A.R.E.

Who Was Edgar Cayce?

Edgar Cayce (1877–1945) was born on a farm near Hopkinsville, Ky. He was an average individual in most respects. Yet, throughout his life, he manifested one of the most remarkable psychic talents of all time. As a young man, he found that he was able to enter into a self–induced trance state, which enabled him to place his mind in contact with an unlimited source of information. While asleep, he could answer questions or give accurate discourses on any topic. These discourses, more than 14,000 in number, were transcribed as he spoke and are called "readings."

Given the name and location of an individual anywhere in the world, he could correctly describe a person's condition and outline a regimen of treatment. The consistent accuracy of his diagnoses and the effectiveness of the treatments he prescribed made him a medical phenomenon, and he came to be called the "father of holistic medicine."

Eventually, the scope of Cayce's readings expanded to include such subjects as world religions, philosophy, psychology, parapsychology, dreams, history, the missing years of Jesus, ancient civilizations, soul growth, psychic development, prophecy, and reincarnation.

A.R.E. Membership

People from all walks of life have discovered meaningful and life–transforming insights through membership in A.R.E. To learn more about Edgar Cayce's A.R.E. and how membership in the A.R.E. can enhance your life, visit our Web site at EdgarCayce.org, or call us toll-free at 800–333–4499.

Edgar Cayce's A.R.E.
215 67th Street
Virginia Beach, VA 23451–2061

EDGARCAYCE.ORG